"This book is a must-read for m
prostate cancer — and their families."

Paul Johnson, M.D.
Chief of Surgery at Ballard
Community Hospital, retired
Seattle, WA

"This book will reward anyone searching for answers
and options for treatment of their prostate cancer. It provides the reader with the tools to become an intregral part
of the decision making process. I highly recommend it."

Michael J. Dattoli, M.D.
University Community Hospital
Tampa, FL

"What a great book you wrote — *Prostate Cancer: A
Survivor's Guide!* I absolutely commend you for doing this
work. This should be required reading for every man older
than 40. A book like yours at the time of my diagnosis
would have been a marvelous find."

Ken Humphrey

"I was diagnosed in January of 1994 . . . and your
book has helped to relieve a lot of my anxiety. It's the best
I've read, and I know it will help others."

Don Cox

"As one who has experienced prostate cancer firsthand,
in his excellent book Don Kaltenbach insightfully describes
what it is like to cope with the disease, and provides other
prostate cancer patients with up-to-date information on both
conventional and investigational therapies currently available."

Norm Jones, M.D.
Director of Radiation Oncology
Piedmont Hospital
Atlanta, GA

PROSTATE CANCER:
A Survivor's Guide

PROSTATE CANCER:
A Survivor's Guide

Don Kaltenbach
with Tim Richards

Seneca House Press
New Port Richey, Florida
BookWorld Services
Sarasota, Florida

Prostate Cancer: A Survivor's Guide
Copyright © 1995 by Don Kaltenbach

Published by Seneca House Press, New Port Richey, Florida.

ISBN: 0-9640088-1-5

Distributor to the trade in the United States: BookWorld Services, Inc., 1933 Whitfield Loop, Sarasota, Florida 34243 (800-444-2524)

Library of Congress Catalog Card Number: 94-121-397

Cover design by Dan Van Loon

Printed by Marrakesh Express, Tarpon Springs, Florida

To my wife, Nancy,
and our three children,
David, Graham, and Whitney,
for their love and support.

Acknowledgments

I am very grateful to a number of people who have contributed to this book, in a variety of ways:

My thanks to the physicians who reviewed this book, for their time and the contribution of their expertise: Dr. Paul Johnson, a surgeon for over 40 years and fellow cancer survivor; Dr. Norm Jones, Director of Radiation Oncology at Piedmont Hospital in Atlanta; and Dr. John Blasko, a leading authority on brachytherapy, for his time, research data, and the fine foreward he wrote for this book.

Chris Jacobs, president of Theragenics, has been a source of support and encouragement from the very beginning. This book has been much enhanced by her help and guidance. I am also indebted to Lloyd Ney, founder of PAACT, for his aid in this endeavor.

I am deeply grateful to TAP Pharmaceuticals, Inc., for their permission to use their fine artwork.

My thanks also to Joanne Denton and Greg Lawrence, for their unceasing efforts on behalf of this project.

Finally, I owe a special debt of gratitude to the late Dr. Harold McDonald. A true professional and southern gentleman, Dr. McDonald was devoted to the practice of medicine and always showed deep concern for his patients. May there be more like him.

CONTENTS

FOREWORD

Over the past decade, the numbers of men diagnosed with prostate cancer have been steadily increasing. As if by stealth, prostate cancer has become the most common form of malignancy and second leading cause of cancer death among American males. It has taken the life of such notables as actors Bill Bixby and Telly Savalas, producer Joseph Papp, and musician Frank Zappa.

Although the disease is both common and serious, it has received little public attention and even less research funding compared to more publicized forms of cancer such as breast cancer. Because prostate cancer is intimately related to male sexuality, many men find the subject embarrassing and are reluctant to talk about it. As a consequence, although any man who lives long enough runs a significant risk of developing prostate cancer, knowledge of the nature and treatment of the disease is as foreign to most men as the principles of quantum mechanics. When confronted with the news that they have prostate cancer, most men are caught utterly unprepared.

In my 15 year career as a Radiation Oncologist, I have been privileged to guide and support thousands of cancer patients and their families through the challenge of cancer. I have witnessed first-hand the full spectrum of human emotion experienced by these patients in their struggle to understand and come to grips with the realities of their disease.

During the last 9 years, my interests have led me to prostate cancer research and treatment. As a result, I have personally counseled and treated over 1000 men who were diagnosed with prostate cancer and faced the difficult task of dealing with the disease on an emotional and physical level. Many men, either by their basic nature, a fear of the unknown, or a sense of being overwhelmed by their diagnosis will unquestioningly accept the prognosis and suggested treatment of their physician. A rare few are unwilling to passively accept their doctor's judgment. They seek to become fully informed about their disease and its treatment so that they may enter into a partnership with their physician to determine what course of action is appropriate for them. It is these patients that come through their treatment more educated and optimistic, with a calming sense of having made the treatment decision that is right for them.

However, the patient who chooses to open this Pandora's box must be prepared for frustration, anxiety and effort. He will be faced with a bewildering array of options and sharply divided opinions about what treatment is best or even whether treatment is necessary. I know of no disease that generates more honest differences of opinion among knowledgeable experts than does prostate cancer. The seeker of knowledge must be prepared for contradictory advice when traveling this road. The work is hard but the rewards immense.

Don Kaltenbach was just such a questioning patient, and his own efforts to inform himself led to the production of this book. His story is a common one, although his treatment decision remains uncommon today. As Don discovered, in the surgical world of urology, radical prostatectomy, or total surgical removal of the prostate, is considered the standard of treatment for early stage prostate cancer. Likewise, in the world of radiation therapy, a series of external beam radiation treatments is often proposed as equally effective. However, modern testing methods now bring into question the effectiveness of both of these methods of treatment. In addition, serious complications of surgery and external beam radiation may dramatically impact the patient's quality of life, and should be weighed against the potential benefits.

The concern over complications influenced Don's own choice of treatment. He chose to avoid surgery and external beam radiation. Instead, he opted for a promising new treatment involving the placement of radioactive implants directly into the prostate. This form of treatment, known as brachytherapy, results in an intense but highly confined dose of radiation to the prostate while sparing the surrounding healthy tissue. Early results of this method indicate an effectiveness equal to that of surgery or traditional external beam radiation, but with a markedly reduced chance of complications. My own experience with this method of treatment over the past 9 years indicates that this procedure offers a real alternative for many men who wish to seek a cure for their disease while minimizing complications.

Don's choice may not be your own. Regardless of what treatment you decide is best for you, this book will prove to be an invaluable resource for you and your family. Don cuts through the confusion surrounding prostate cancer, and provides an honest and up-to-date evaluation of all the available treatment options.

The emotional burden of dealing with a cancer diagnosis is often more difficult than coping with the physical impact of the disease. Don deals with the emotional aspects of prostate cancer in a way few physicians can — from personal experience. Having been there himself, he understands the vital concerns of the patient. His advice and encouragement will be a boon to fellow cancer sufferers as they come to terms with their disease.

An educated and insightful patient such as Don Kaltenbach is a great value not only to others who share his condition, but also to the medical community. Often, because our training emphasizes the treatment of diseases, we physicians may forget that we must treat the patient, not just the disease. We must listen to and appreciate the attitudes and desires of the patient, who will have to live with the consequences of our treatment. Don's views and choices, carefully elucidated, provide a corrective to physicians who may be prone to be overly rigid in their approach to treatment. Don reminds us that even doctors can still learn a thing or two.

So, if you or a loved one is confronted with the diagnosis of prostate cancer and you wish to begin your own journey of discovery, I can think of no better guidebook than **Prostate Cancer: A Survivor's Guide.**

John C. Blasko, M.D.
Northwest Tumor Institute
Seattle, WA

DIVIDED HIGHWAY
BEGINS

INTRODUCTION: THE JOURNEY AHEAD

"Not I, not anyone else can travel that road for you. You must travel it for yourself."

Walt Whitman

Much of the information available within this book can be found in other sources, in booklets and pamphlets describing prostate cancer, in articles and medical journals. Yet in many instances, easily accessible information on the nature of prostate cancer and the alternatives the patient possesses for treating the disease is sadly lacking. This is particularly tragic in the case of prostate cancer, a common disease among men the treatment of which has seen tremendous advances in recent years. But the patient who remains uninformed of these advances, and the spawning of new treatment alternatives, cannot hope to benefit from them. The primary goal of this book is to provide this information to the prostate cancer patient.

Prostate cancer is more than a technical description of a disease and its available treatments. It is a journey. Four years ago, I made this journey, from discovery to recovery. It is my hope that reading this account of my own experiences will provide you with an expectation of what your own journey might hold for you.

In this sense, by calling this book "a survivor's guide," I mean more than a source of useful information. I myself am a survivor, who has made the difficult passage from one side to the other. My hope is that this book will provide direction for those who also must come this way, to make the road easier and the destination more sure.

Chapter 1

DISCOVERY

*"Last night I dreamt I was in the labyrinth,
And woke far on. I did not know the place."*

Edwin Muir

No matter how you try to prepare, life will surprise you. Without surprises, life would not have its excitement or its unexpected griefs, its hopes or its fears. Each day is a process of discovery, a dawning of new challenges. Many of life's surprises we adapt to readily: we change a plan, adjust our routine. We take them in stride and go on.

But some of life's surprises come at us from out of nowhere. Some shake our world. The year of 1990 held such a surprise in store for me.

The year of '89 had already seen dramatic changes in my life. After working as a lawyer in New Port Richey, Florida for almost two decades, I had begun building a new office. Not only that, my wife Nancy and I had a new baby on the way.

Nancy and I had been trying for years to have a baby, unsuccessfully. Eventually, we both went through testing to find out if something was wrong. When we were told we couldn't have any children, we decided to adopt. We adopted David in 1985, and planned to adopt a second little boy, Graham, in 1988.

It may have been the very week we brought Graham home that Nancy became pregnant! This was an unexpected joy for us after years of frustration. In July of 1989, Nancy gave birth to a little girl, Whitney. Ironically, this undeniable proof that I was fertile led Nancy to suggest I have a vasectomy. So on her birthday, November 10th, I went to a local urologist and had the operation. We had friends over and had a birthday party highlighted by a mock vasectomy performed behind a backlit screen. Happy birthday, honey!

A couple of months later I noticed a little blood in my urine. Although I felt no pain or discomfort, I immediately called the urologist who had performed my vasectomy. The doctor suspected it was an infection from the operation and prescribed some antibiotics. Two weeks went by, but the problem didn't clear up. So I went in to see the doctor.

He ordered an ultrasound, a diagnostic technique known in the medical journals as "transrectal ultrasonography," or TRUS for short (don't be alarmed --- you won't need one after the procedure). The sound waves produced by the instrument echo off internal organs of the body and produce an image on a little TV monitor. From what I could make of it, the screen could have been showing anything from the air traffic at O'Hare to an old monochrome video game, but to the doctor's trained eye, it was a map of my body's interior. Almost immediately, he detected a spot on my prostate, and pointed it out to me: a bright patch on the screen about the size of a dime.

Later, he performed a biopsy, guiding a needle probe with the ultrasound to take samples from the prostate. He took six samples. The probe didn't hurt particularly; a lot of the discomfort is psychological rather than physical. Many individuals suffer considerable anxiety over these tests, whether it be from the invasion or the associated discomfort. But they are really less appalling than we imagine, and are truly invaluable for accurate diagnosis. After a while, you get used to it, and it all becomes very matter of course. Take my word for it.

After the tests, I went home. The spot on my prostate bothered me a bit, but I didn't really think too much about it. The doctor hadn't said much during the biopsy, and so I felt I had little need to be overly concerned. He told me he would be sending the samples to the lab for examination, and would get back to me with the results in about ten days. So I just went back about my business, and thought no more about it.

Ten days later, a call came in at my office. Rather than tell me the results of the biopsy over the phone, the doctor wanted to see me in person. It was my first intimation that something was definitely wrong.

I dropped by the urologist's office, uncertain of what awaited me. I was seated in a small room, and the doctor came in with the results of my biopsy in a folder. He didn't look at me, but instead kept his eyes on his watch, as though pressed for time.

In a matter-of-fact tone of voice, he said, "You've got cancer, and we have to operate. We can give you a penile implant."

I was dumbstruck. What little else he told me I remember only vaguely, for my mind was in a fog. Even with the advance warnings, it somehow came to me as a shock. I had cancer. The big C.

We all have some conception of how our lives are to play out. We may not know exactly what cards we'll be dealt, but we have an idea, an image of our future. Yet the news I had just received had in one moment eclipsed my view of the future, and threatened to blot out the life I had always envisioned for myself.

I was told I would have to return for some additional tests to see if the cancer had spread beyond the prostate. I nodded dumbly. I didn't even think to ask any questions about my condition.

I walked out of that office with nothing. Not even a brochure. I had been told I had prostate cancer, but that meant nothing to me. All I knew was what we all know, that cancer kills.

That evening I went to my racquetball club, and pounded a ball off the wall. Whack. Whack. Whack. It seemed unimaginable what was happening to me. I was forty-four. I had a beautiful wife and three young children, two of them still in diapers. The words of an associate flashed into my mind. He'd told me he had lost his father when he was four. Would my children grow up without a father?

Yet I felt fine. As I pounded on the racquetball, it seemed to me I felt as good as ever. How could I be dying? I wondered if somehow a mistake had been made. A misdiagnosis. A slip-up at the lab. Something.

When you make a terrible discovery such as this, the mind turns over and over, and oscillates from one extreme to another, as though trapped in a maze. I had always been a strong, resourceful individual, but suddenly I found myself in unknown territory. I was lost.

A Common Problem

What I didn't know then, and have since learned, is just how many men find themselves in this same situation. In 1994, approximately 200,000 men were diagnosed with prostate cancer in the U.S. In the same year, approximately 38,000 died from from the disease. On an average day, about 550 men will be told for the first time, as I was, that they have prostate cancer.

Although prostate cancer is very rare among men under 50, it becomes more prevalent with age. With men 65 or older, there is an 80% chance of acquiring the disease, although most of these men may never know they possess the disease. And since the U.S. contains a rapidly aging population, the problem is on the rise. In the last five years, the number of men diagnosed with prostate cancer has doubled, and some believe the disease will soon reach epidemic proportions.

Yet few men are aware of the threat. Up until recently, prostate cancer has been largely neglected in the media as a medical issue. Perhaps due to the lack of attention it has received, research on prostate cancer is significantly underfunded, relative to other common forms of cancer. For instance, the National Cancer Institute, a major source of cancer research funding, spends almost six times as much on breast cancer, a women's disease comparable in incidence and severity to prostate cancer in men.

The good news is that the prognosis for those who develop prostate cancer has greatly improved in recent years. The last decade has seen dramatic advances made in the treatment of the disease. Regardless of the stage the cancer has progressed to, now more than ever, there is real reason for hope.

The key is to learn about your options. At first, every man diagnosed with prostate cancer will find himself where I was: lost and in the dark. From that there is no escape. But there is a way through, there is hope for tomorrow.

After the first traumatic discovery of cancer, the temptation is to hide from the truth. But discovery is an ally. The knowledge you gain, now and in the future, can be your guide through that dark passage from cancer victim to cancer survivor.

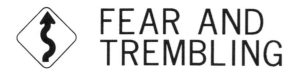 FEAR AND TREMBLING

"My heart is in anguish within me;
the terrors of death assail me.
Fear and trembling have beset me;
horror has overwhelmed me;
I said, 'Oh, that I had the wings of a dove!
I would fly away and be at rest —
I would flee far away ...'"

Psalms 55:4-7

For the first few days, I told no one about my secret. Not my friends, not my associates, not even my wife. I felt I needed some time to come to grips with the situation on my own.

In the meantime, I threw myself into my work. Construction on my law office was close to completion, and when I wasn't involved with a client, I kept myself occupied with the selection of carpets and wallpaper, colors and furnishings for the various rooms. The work was therapeutic, and allowed me to turn my attention to things other than my recent diagnosis.

But in the back of my mind, the problem continued to grind away. At moments, the nagging feeling would rush to the forefront, and I would be confronted with questions about what my condition meant, and what my future held.

Interrogations of the Heart

Though I did not realize it at the time, the questions I was asking myself reflected many of the emotional reactions any individual goes through upon diagnosis with cancer. The questions we ask ourselves can also tell us a lot about the way we try to cope with our cancer. The following are some of the questions I found continually returning to my mind — in all likelihood, they will be familiar to every individual faced with this dilemma.

"How could this be happening to me?"

The immediate reaction of anyone who learns they have cancer will be shock and disbelief. Often, this reaction will endure long after the discovery stage. The feeling may also reemerge again and again throughout the ups and downs of testing and treatment. Moments of panic and uncertainty are normal and to be expected in anyone faced with cancer and its consequences. For men with prostate cancer, there is not only the threat of death, but of intimacy-ending side-effects that seem almost as frightening. Dealing with cancer can leave you feeling that your life has been turned upside down, with no hope to make things right again.

The sense that your life is coming apart can leave you confused and unable to concentrate, or paralyzed and unable to act. The emotions that overtake us at this time may seem strange and unnatural, but they are typical of anyone going through a traumatic experience. I myself felt as though the unimaginable had happened, as though I'd been hit by a meteor. I'd always thought of cancer as a disease that afflicts the old, yet I was only in my early forties. I had three young children. How could I have cancer?

It is always a struggle to find a way to cope with the impact of disease. Underlying the question "How could this be happening to me?" and all the emotions that accompany it, we are really asking ourselves, "How do I make sense of and cope with what has happened to me?" It is the first step in our struggle, a step we may need to retrace many times along the way.

At times it may seem there is no answer to the question, but don't give up. When you feel panic, remind yourself of some important facts.

- Your body does not hate you. Life does not hate you. God does not hate you. You have a disease.

- Prostate cancer is not synonymous with death. You have every reason to believe you will survive this ordeal.

- There are many available treatments to successfully combat the disease.

- There is no reason to expect permanent side-effects, and if there are any, they can be controlled or mitigated.

- You can control the process of living with, treating, and overcoming your cancer.

- Cancer can open up positive avenues of change in your life, whether they be emotional, relational or spiritual.

"I feel good. How could I have cancer?"

The desire to avoid facing a painful truth can be overwhelming at times. When an individual's thoughts or perceptions do not conform to reality, but instead are attempts to escape from it, he is said to be "in denial." And no matter how clearheaded the individual, he is almost certain to experience some degree of denial once confronted with the grim reality of cancer. Even physicians who have treated cancer patients struggle with denial when they are themselves diagnosed with the dread disease.

Denial is a defense mechanism. It allows us to avoid or block out information which we are psychologically unable to absorb all at once. And denial can manifest itself in a variety of ways. Frequently, a patient, when first informed of his cancer by his doctor, will fail to understand or later recall the details of his diagnosis. Some will avoid talking about the illness and pretend as if it didn't exist. Still others will be unrealistically optimistic, refusing to accept the seriousness of their illness or expecting a sudden, miraculous cure. All of these are symptomatic of someone in denial.

Denial can be a blessing when it protects us from excessive anxiety or depression. A short vacation from a world of troubles can be a restorative for the mind and body. But reality has a way of catching up with those that run from it, and severe denial has a variety of harmful consequences. It may keep the individual from seeking proper medical treatment. Even if it doesn't interfere with his treatment, denial can distort his personal relationships and obstruct open and honest communication with friends and family members.

Most who get prostate cancer will pass through a period of denial, and gradually come to an acceptance of their condition. For me many weeks passed before I surrendered my doubts concerning my diagnosis with cancer. I don't think I came to fully accept I had prostate cancer until my operation months later. Fortunately, these doubts did not interfere with my attempts to deal responsibly with the problem. I have heard of others who were not so fortunate. Recently, a friend told me about a local man who refused to believe he had prostate cancer. Time passed and eventually the disease spread throughout his body. Now he is in the latter stages of the disease. He's terminal, but he still remains convinced he has nothing but a bad case of the flu! It's okay to have doubts or suspicions about what a doctor tells you, but don't let it keep you from getting more information or finding good medical care. Your life may depend on it.

"Why me?"

After the initial shock, depression will almost certainly follow. Weeping, despair, a sense of guilt, all these are symptoms of depression and are completely normal. Men often feel that tears are a sign of weakness, or that we should be tough and stand up to the disease, rather than succomb to melancholy. But who would say to someone who is overcome with grief at the loss of a loved one, "Buck up! Be a man and stop your moping!" In a way, the prospects confronting someone with cancer are far worse: the loss of life, of the future, of his loved ones, of everything he cherishes.

It is understandable that one should become depressed at such losses. If you have prostate cancer, don't punish yourself for feeling down. The presence of those who care about you can be a comfort. Prayer too can lift your spirits, even in sorrow. If you know someone who has this disease and is gripped by depression, you need not always try to cheer them up or talk them out of being sad. The best response is simply to be there for that person, to be understanding and sympathetic.

"Will I lose my family?"

This was my greatest fear, greater than the fear of death itself. The idea that my children might grow up without their father really got to me. As in my case, the fear of death is often accompanied or even overshadowed by other fears and anxieties. Among them are: fear of pain, fear of impairment or humiliation, fear of being a burden, fear of being alone or deserted, and fear of financial difficulties due to the costs of medical treatment.

A time of crisis will bring out in us a myriad of fears and inadequacies that would otherwise remain hidden and unknown. These added insecurities can weigh us down, and greatly magnify the stress we feel as we seek to manage not only our cancer but its impact on every aspect of our lives.

At times the burden may seem too much to bear, so don't try to bear it all on your own. Rely on the support of family and friends, and share your apprehensions with them. You may find it helpful to turn to your local church for spiritual guidance and financial aid. Hospitals will sometimes provide counseling for cancer outpatients in need of emotional support. Also, there are support groups for those with cancer and their families (*see Appendix A: Where to Get Help*).

At the same time, it is important that you not dwell on your problems to the extent that they leave you feeling helpless. You are not helpless. Determine what things you can do, and set realistic goals for yourself. Only you can take responsibility for directing your cancer treatment, so become informed, seek out good medical care, and look after your health. Avoid fixating on your problems by keeping yourself active. Work and exercise were both helpful to me in keeping a sense of order to life and taking my mind off my problems. If you still work, make it business as usual as best you can. Social activities can serve as a valuable outlet as well. At times you may not feel like doing any of these things, but your emotional well-being has an impact on your health. Look at it as part of your medical treatment.

"Can anyone know what I'm going through?"

Most cancer patients experience some degree of isolation as a consequence of their disease. Many report feeling separated or different from others. The mere fact of the illness becomes an invisible barrier between the sufferer and other people.

There are really two sources for this sense of isolation. The first comes from within the person suffering from cancer. Internal feelings and emotions may act to drive him away from others. He may feel strange, uncomfortable or embarrassed in the presence of others. He may withdraw and feel a desire to be alone. I know that when something is bothering me, I have a tendency to become quiet and withdraw into myself. It's a common reaction.

The other source of isolation comes from the outside: the social stigma attached to cancer, or any serious illness, in our society. Ours is a culture that prizes health and well-being, and displays an unnatural fear of illness and death. We keep sick people in hospitals, away from the rest of society, thus enabling us to avoid the difficult issues of sickness and mortality. In a sense, our whole society may be said to be in denial over death.

This cultural bias is reflected in the attitudes of individuals toward the sick. They often don't know what to say or how to act around the sick person, and feel discomfort being near him. Even loved ones may respond this way. Many avoid the sick person, because he is a reminder that cancer can strike anyone. They turn a blind eye to the illness, and tell themselves. "It can't happen to me."

Before my cancer, I would hear of someone who had it and say that it was a shame. But although I could express sympathy for others with cancer, I did not really know how to relate to them or their ordeal. You have to go through it yourself, and once you do, it is as if your eyes are opened. Cancer becomes real and personal to you, and suddenly you understand just how they felt. Most people are like me. Until they have felt the personal impact of cancer on their own lives, they will not be able to truly identify with your situation.

You may even sense that people treat you differently, which can intensify your sense of isolation, and leave you feeling alone in your fight against the disease. If you do feel isolated, find someone you can trust to open up to and express how you're feeling. This may be a family member, friend, counselor, or another victim of cancer. Appendix A of this book provides a list of cancer support groups formed to offer this kind of support to individuals with cancer.

These are only a few of the questions that we who have prostate cancer will ask ourselves. Behind the questions seethe a host of powerful emotions: fear, anger, confusion, self-pity, bitterness, despair, and others. Doctors can help the body in its battle against the cancer inside, but they can do little to help the patient in his fight to come to grips with the emotional and psychological impacts of prostate cancer. At the same time, there is a growing awareness in the medical community of the important role the patient's emotions have in his recovery. Negative emotions can weaken the immune system, but a positive attitude can aid it in its fight.

Thus, in a way, half the battle is up to you. Although a positive mental attitude cannot cure you in and of itself, it can improve the body's response to medical treatment. But don't think if you do have periods of anxiety, anger, or depression that you have failed, or are somehow "making yourself worse." Anyone who suffers from cancer will struggle with these feelings from time to time. The important thing is to not succumb to them.

Opposite these negative emotions are positive emotions and attitudes that can strenghthen you. Courage, confidence, amusement, serenity, joy in the little things in life, and, above all, hope. Cultivate these. They are your weapons as you close for battle with the enemy.

Breaking the Silence

The first week after my diagnosis was a difficult time. Members of my staff, who are very much like a family to me, noticed I was very quiet and withdrawn. Eventually, one of my secretaries came into my office and asked me if something was wrong. I didn't even want to pronounce the word — I just said I had the big C.

By the end of the week, I decided I needed to tell Nancy. I had an appointment to see the urologist for follow-up tests within a few days, and I wanted her to go with me. My wife is a very supportive person, and I knew, whatever happened, that I could depend on her. But when the moment of truth arrived, I didn't know quite what to say. I just mumbled, "I've got prostate cancer," and left it at that. She was very concerned, but took the news with characteristic quiet strength. Later she would tell me it was the most depressed she had ever seen me.

Normally, she would call close friends and family when she needed someone to talk to, but I asked her to keep it to herself for a while. She found it very hard to hold in such a revelation, but for my sake agreed.

Then we went to a bookstore to see if we could find any information on prostate cancer. For a week I had been set adrift by what had befallen me. Now it was time to start taking action.

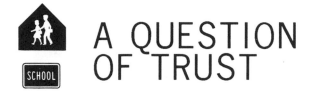 A QUESTION
OF TRUST

"Know the truth, and the truth shall set you free."

John 8:32

In March, I returned to the doctor for a bone scan and CT scan, to check for the spread of cancer beyond the prostate. These tests are part of what is known as a "metastatic workup," and are used to determine the stage to which the cancer has advanced.

During the previous two weeks, I had done some research on prostate cancer, and had managed to find out a little more about my condition and the tests I would be undergoing.

When prostate cancer metastasizes (spreads beyond the original site of the tumor), it usually settles into the lymph nodes or bones. The bone scan is used to examine the nearby bones of the back, hips and legs for the presence of the cancer. On the other hand, the CT scan is used to examine the soft tissues: the lymph nodes, the lungs, and the prostate itself.

Early in the morning, a mildly radioactive liquid was injected into a vein in my right arm. I left with the instruction to go drink a lot of liquids, and returned later in the day for my bone scan. Once in the bloodstream, the radioactive substance worked its way through my body to settle in the bones. When I returned to the doctor's office, I was told to lay down on a table, and a plate was lowered down over my head. The plate was part of a machine called a "scanner." As the plate slowly moved down toward my toes, the scanner recorded an image of my body. Because areas of bone infected with cancer tend to absorb more of the radioactive material than normal bone, any bone cancer will appear as bright spots on the film. A bone scan is far more sensitive than a typical x-ray for revealing bone cancer, and although bone damage, arthritis, and some other conditions may also show up as bright patches on the scan, a trained specialist will usually be able to distinguish the difference.

The CT scan (or CAT scan) uses "computerized tomography" to give a three-dimensional view inside the body. The arm of the scanner directs pinpoint-thin x-ray beams through the portions of the body under examination as it rapidly passes over you. Each pass provides a cross-section of the body's internal structures, and as many as eight scans per centimeter are taken. The data is

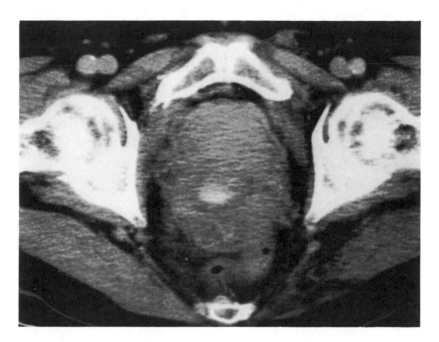

Figure 1. This is a CT scan of a prostate gland. The prostate shows significant enlargement due to the presence of extensive cancer.

fed into a minicomputer, which converts the information into a three-dimensional image. The image gives a more precise and accurate picture of the internal organs than the flat view provided by a conventional x-ray, which superimposes overlapping organs and can only dimly represent the soft tissues of the body.

I went to a radiologist for this test. Because of its size, the CT scan machine commands an entire room. I laid down on a table inside a big tube. Because it was quite cold, they covered me with a blanket. I underwent a series of scans of my lower abdomen, taken from different angles. The entire process took about half an hour, during which I had to remain completely still. There was, however, no discomfort, and although it seems like a long time to receive external radiation, I'm told that the CAT scan actually exposes the patient to no more radiation than a normal x-ray. And the nuclear tracers used in the bone scan are not only very weak, but pass out of the body within 48 hours.

About a week later, the doctor discussed the results of the tests with Nancy and me. As before, he was brief and appeared hurried. He indicated that the tests showed no spread of the cancer beyond the prostate, but again strongly urged that I have the cancer cut out as soon as possible.

I was greatly relieved to hear the cancer was still contained, but I still didn't feel I knew enough about my condition to make an informed decision. I was told I would be in the hospital for seven to ten days and laid up for another six to eight weeks. He had impressed upon me the urgency of my situation. I needed to have the operation before further spread of the cancer. That scared me. But the potential consequences of the operation were also frightening. I would probably be impotent, and might suffer from incontinence, not to mention the potential danger of the operation itself. Jack, a good friend and neighbor of mine, had recently had a radical prostatectomy. He had hemorrhaged on the table and almost died. I just wasn't sure what to do. One book I had read suggested that any patient considering a major operation should get a second opinion. So I asked the doctor for a referral.

"You can go to the Moffitt Cancer Center in Tampa," he said. "But we're just as good as they are, and besides, we're closer."

After leaving his office, I still felt dissatisfied. Nancy, who is usually far more tolerant than I, was even more displeased with the doctor's manner. We decided I should at least go to the Moffitt Center, which was only an hour's drive away, before making any crucial decisions.

A few days later, I spoke to a family doctor I knew. I told him about my condition and described how the local urologist had pressed me to have the surgery.

"Wow!" he said. "That seems a little severe to insist on immediately cutting it out."

His statement confirmed a suspicion that had been growing in me for some time.

"Where else should I go?" I asked.

He told me he would be glad to check around for me, and find alternative sites that were well equipped to treat prostate cancer. He returned with a list of four places where I could go. Among them were Duke University Hospital, located on the North Carolina campus, and Johns Hopkins Hospital in Baltimore.

After some consideration, I set up an appointment at Johns Hopkins Hospital, and arranged to fly up to Baltimore. But first I would stop by the Moffitt Center in Tampa.

The director of the Moffitt Center treated Nancy and me very well. He spoke to us at length and provided us with additional materials that gave specific information on prostate cancer and available methods of treatment. The director suggested two possible options for my case: radiation therapy or a radical prostatectomy. He recommended the latter. As many as half of all men who undergo a radical prostatectomy will become impotent as a result of the operation, and occasionally there is a subsequent bladder control problem as well. But because I was still young, his prognosis was very favorable in my case. His optimism relieved a great deal of my anxiety concerning the prostatectomy and its side-effects, but part of me was still hoping I wouldn't need the operation.

I had been reading through a cancer handbook, and one of the suggested options for prostate cancer was to do nothing at all. I suggested to the director that I actually had a third option: to wait, and undergo no treatment at all for the time being.

He listened thoughtfully, but pointed out that I was still only in my forties, and the cancer would in all likelihood continue to grow. It might be years before the cancer caused further complications, but sooner or later it would catch up with me.

"One day," he said, "You're going to hop off the plane and your leg is going to break, because cancer has gotten into your bones."

I realized he was right. It would be irresponsible of me to wait and do nothing, and in the end I would suffer the consequences of my choice. I needed to take care of the problem before it was too late.

It was early May when Nancy and I took off from Florida in my Piper Seneca. The weather was clear for most of the flight, but there was heavy cloud cover over Baltimore. The fog was as thick as soup all the way down on our approach to the airport — until about 200 feet, when we broke through and could see the landing strip stretched out before us. I hoped it was a good omen. Maybe I would also break through the fog of uncertainty that I had been enduring now that I had arrived in Baltimore.

I had reason to be optimistic. By chance, that very week an article had appeared in *The U.S. News & World Report* magazine (April 30, 1990) that rated the finest hospitals in the country. The article recommended that a man diagnosed with prostate cancer should find care in a leading institution. Doctors were surveyed to determine the best hospitals for each of twelve specialties. I saw that Johns Hopkins had been selected by more doctors than any other hospital in the specialty of urology. Furthermore, the article mentioned a new nerve-sparing technique used in prostate surgery that significantly reduced the likelihood of impotence. The procedure was pioneered by Dr. Patrick Walsh, chief of urology at Johns Hopkins. My confidence was growing that there might be a happy resolution after all.

After stopping at the hotel, we made our way to Johns Hopkins Hospital. There we met with a third-year resident, who assisted Dr. Walsh in the Urology department.

"I know you're only here for a second opinion," he said. "But this is a great hospital."

He suggested that instead of having the operation performed in Florida, I have the operation at Johns Hopkins instead. He made sense. Everything I had learned confirmed that the Urology department at Johns Hopkins was very possibly the best place in the country for the treatment of prostate cancer. But I still wanted to weigh my options.

"You know," he continued. "You really should do something about this rather than just gather information and put it off. This operation will work for you."

He convinced me to sign up for an operation, scheduled for August 6th, the earliest available date. Although Nancy would have supported me no matter what I chose to do, she was very pleased with my decision. My head told me it was the best thing to do, but I still had some reservations. I felt healthy, and that puzzled me. Also, Jack's close call on the operating table, and his post-operative problems came back to mind. If I could find a reasonable alternative, I still hoped to avoid going through with the operation.

As we were preparing to leave, I asked the resident, "By the way, I had my medical reports sent up here. Have you gotten a look at them yet?"

"No," he replied.

"Well," I asked. "What makes you think I need to have this operation?"

He didn't really have an answer, and that troubled me.

It continued to trouble me even after I flew back to Florida, and returned to my work. Instead of a sense of confidence that my problem would soon be taken care of, I struggled with growing doubts. Every one of the doctors I had seen were pushing me to have the operation. Each argued that, for different reasons, I should have it done at their medical facility. The resident at Johns Hopkins had done the same, without even looking at my test results! How could he have known what was in my best interest without any examination of my particular case?

Perhaps I'm just suspicious by nature, but it dawned on me that the resident may not have been serving my interests so much as the economic interests of the hospital, or his own desire to gain further surgical experience.

I wanted to believe the doctors I had seen, but I wasn't certain I had been told the whole truth. Did I know all the facts? Did I know all my options? In the end, I wasn't sure who I should trust.

Finding the Right Doctor

If you are like most people, finding a family doctor that you like and trust is important. But if it is important to find such a doctor to treat the common ailments that occasionally visit us all, it is critical that you find a physician you truly trust when faced with a life-threatening disease like cancer.

Yet few make a carefully reasoned decision when it comes to selecting a physician to guide their cancer treatment. Usually, the diagnosis is made as part of a regular physical exam, or is found while investigating the cause of an ailment. In either instance, the discovery of cancer comes as a surprise.

While still numb from the shock, the patient is referred by the diagnosing doctor to a nearby specialist. If the patient is in a hospital, he may be sent to a specialist in a different department at the hospital. If the doctor belongs to a group practice, the patient may be referred to one of the doctor's associates. If the doctor is himself a specialist, he may take over the patient's care personally. In any case, the patient typically finds himself in the care of a doctor he had a very limited role in choosing.

Like many people, you may find it difficult to leave the care of the doctor who initiated your treatment. But there is really no reason to feel obligated to a particular physician. If a doctor is not right for you, find another. You need not even provide the doctor with a reason for your decision to leave his care.

Cancer not only demands that you find a doctor that you have confidence in, it also demands much of your doctor as well. As described in the previous chapter, cancer not only has a physical impact that must be treated, but a dramatic effect on your thoughts and emotions as well. The physician who treats cancer patients should be aware of their special needs and be capable of establishing a therapeutic doctor-patient relationship. Such a doctor will make the road to recovery easier and less stressful for you.

If you are considering whether you should stay under the care of your present physician, or if you're actively searching for the right doctor to direct your prostate cancer treatment, consider the following questions:

Is the doctor respected by his/her colleagues?

A number of objective criteria can be used to help you evaluate a doctor's merit. A doctor with staff priveleges at one or more hospitals will have usually demonstrated the necessary surgical proficiency and good judgment to earn the respect of his or her colleagues. Review-committee membership at a respected medical institution also indicates a doctor's reputation among his or her peers. A doctor whose practice is hospital-based or part of a group practice is to be preferred, since any reputable hospital or group practice will require their physicians undergo peer review sufficient to ensure quality care.

The kind of hospital the doctor is affiliated with is also relevant. A doctor on staff at a university or medical school hospital is more likely to be in good standing in the medical community. To a lesser degree, this also applies to doctors with membership at a large community hospital.

It is advisable to find a doctor who treats a large number of prostate cancer patients, and is therefore more familiar with the kind of care they require. A physician who works in a National Cancer Institute designated cancer center is more likely to be familiar with the latest developments in cancer treatment.

Any of these criteria will improve one's chances of finding a capable physician, but the best means is probably by referral from a local, trusted doctor who is familiar with the reputable and respected physicians in the area.

Does the doctor have good credentials?

Board certification will indicate that a doctor has been thoroughly examined although it cannot guarantee his competence. Certification in a specialty, especially oncology, or possession of a board fellowship are further evidences of distinction.

It is possible to check the credentials of a doctor with the Directory of Medical Specialists or the American Medical Directory, a copy of which can be found in the reference room of your local library.

A doctor that possesses none of these credentials is not necessarily a bad doctor, but you will need to find other grounds for trusting yourself to his or her care.

Does the doctor communicate well?

A good physician will explain your condition in detail, taking the time to answer all of your questions and correcting any misconceptions you may have. It is your right to receive a complete description of all your options, and their advantages and disadvantages ---- vital information if you are to have a sense of control over what is happening to you. If the doctor fails to disclose this information, or does not encourage you to choose for yourself which treatment you wish to receive, find another doctor.

Throughout the period of your treatment, the physician should continue to keep you fully informed of the nature and rationale behind any tests or procedures recommended to you. Clear and concise written materials that explain the basic facts of prostate cancer, its symptoms and various treatment alternatives, should also be made available.

Does the physician show personal interest in you and your case?

A doctor who communicates concern for the patient as an individual will ease the treatment process. A doctor who cares will inspire trust in his patients and help to allay their fears. A relationship of trust and care between doctor and patient can greatly contribute to the patient's recovery. But a doctor who sees each patient only as another medical condition to treat will leave his patients feeling alienated, confused and anxious. Ultimately, such a doctor will impede the progress of those under his care.

Is the doctor optimistic?

A doctor who expresses belief that you can be successfully treated will be of great advantage to you. Optimism is infectious. If your physician believes in the likelihood of your recovery, he will encourage a positive attitude in you.

Do you feel comfortable with the doctor?

In the final analysis, all of the above questions come down to this. Do you trust and have confidence in your physician? Does he put you at ease? Are you able to talk with your physician in a relaxed manner?

A doctor may be completely suited for treating some patients and unsuited for treating others. It may be nothing more than a matter of incompatible personalities. Yet you will be making some critical decisions with this doctor, and undergoing a treatment process that can be difficult and extend for months or even years. You will need a doctor you can depend on when the going gets tough. If for any reason you do not feel comfortable with your physician, you should carefully consider whether it is in your interests to find care elsewhere.

I simply didn't feel comfortable with my local doctor. He didn't communicate, or seem personally involved in my case. As a consequence, I experienced doubts and suspicion. It occurred to me that my doubts may have been rooted in anxiety over "going under the knife." But regardless of the reason, I lacked confidence in him. So I decided to go elsewhere for treatment.

But even after seeing the doctors at the Moffitt Center and Johns Hopkins Hospital, I felt uncertain. I can be stubborn at times, and I determined to keep searching for alternatives to surgery. I hoped that I might yet find some other solution.

Happily, my hopes were soon to be rewarded.

Chapter 4

🛑 THE ENEMY WITHIN

"The beginning of health is to know the disease."

Cervantes, Don Quixote

The months after my diagnosis with prostate cancer were a time of searching. I gathered as much material as I could find on the topic. I read and reread what I had found, trying to make sense of it all. Each article, newspaper clipping or pamphlet was like a piece to a puzzle. I hoped that, when I finally put all the pieces together, I would know what I had to do.

We all have a natural inclination to learn, to be drawn to that which is mysterious or unknown. They call this inquisitive principle in human nature curiosity. But the more profound and personal the mystery, the greater the intensity of our interest. When it's a matter of life and death, "curiosity" seems too weak a word to describe this need to know. It becomes a compulsion, a quest for answers.

Don't deny this desire for knowledge. Curiosity may have killed the cat, but there's a good chance it can keep you alive. Too often, individuals will push aside this urge to know, opting for the "quick fix," and later come to regret their rush to take the easy way out.

Be realistic. Do not let months and years pass idly while you peruse the entire Library of Congress for tiny scraps of information. At the same time, don't listen to anyone who tells you there's not a moment to lose, and you have no time to learn about your options. Most cases of prostate cancer are slow growing, and no cancer grows so rapidly that you don't have the time to come to an intelligent decision. Take the time to inform yourself. It will be time well spent.

Here is some of what I learned on my own "quest for answers," both prior to and since my recovery from prostate cancer.

What is Cancer?

When in war, as the military dictum states, it is a necessity to "know thy enemy." This applies to cancer as well, a war not of men and nations but of cells within the body. This war within is not an invasion by outside agents, such as viruses or bacteria, but an uprising from inside. Part of the body is in rebellion against the natural order of the system.

Cancer begins in a single cell. Something goes wrong. The cell may be located in virtually any part of the body: the lung, the blood, the colon, the bladder, a woman's breast or a man's prostate. Each type of cell, such as a blood cell or skin cell, possesses particular traits and has a specific function within the body. It has long been known that cancer cells behave differently depending on their site of origin. On this basis, medical science has identified over one hundred distinct forms of cancer, grouped into five categories according to the kind of tissue in which the cancer starts: carcinomas, melanomas, sarcomas, lymphomas, and leukemia (or cancer of the blood). Almost all cases of prostate cancer — those with which this book is concerned — are carcinomas, which arise in tissues that line or cover an organ.

All forms of cancer bear certain similarities. Wherever the malignant cell occurs, the cell's normal function is subverted. It begins to behave abnormally. Among the characteristics of this transformation in the cell is a certain hyperactivity; the cancer cell multiplies uncontrollably, spreading its subversion into the surrounding tissues. Also, the cancer cell loses some or all of the functions of a normal cell, appearing unformed or, as doctors call it, undifferentiated. Scientists believe that such cancer cells occur hundreds or thousands of times within each individual, but the body's policing agency, the immune system, sends antibodies to attack and destroy the cell before it can reproduce.

If the cancer is able to gain a foothold through rapid growth or resistence to the constant assaults of the body's defenses, what started as a single cell will form into a subversive community of cells, called a tumor. All tumors are the product of abnormal growth, but not all tumors are cancerous; in fact, most are benign. Benign tumors seldom pose a significant threat to health. Unlike malignant tumors, they grow at a more moderate rate, and do not destroy healthy cells. The cells of a benign tumor may appear completely normal, and the arrangement of cells form an orderly pattern, similar to the tissues in which the abnormal growth begins.

The malignant tumor, formed of cancer cells, exhibits excessive and unlimited growth. Not only do the individual cells of the malignant tumor appear and behave abnormally, the mass of cells shows irregular organization, and will expand beyond the boundaries of the tissue or organ where the cancer originated. The cells of the tumor divide at a steady rate, doubling in number over a specific period of time. The time it takes a cancer tumor to double in mass differs for each case, and is known as its doubling rate. It can vary from a few days to years. By the time a tumor has grown to the size of a pea, it has doubled about thirty times, and contains in excess of one billion cells.

Another characteristic of most cancerous tumors is the ability to metastasize, or spread to distant sites of the body. Microscopic clumps of cancer cells break away from the original tumor and travel via the bloodstream or lymph system to another location of the body, where new tumors begin to grow. These metastatic tumors, wherever they have formed, are still made of the same kind of cells as the original tumor. Prostate cancer that has spread to the bones does not become bone cancer. It is prostate cancer outside the prostate, and needs to be treated accordingly.

As the cancerous growth expands, it presses on surrounding tissues, and replaces healthy cells at the perimeter of the mass. As it grows in size, symptoms of the disease will begin to appear. These vary depending on the site and nature of the cancer. Although in some cases, the cancer will remain localized, sometimes the cancer will metastisize and spread the disease to other parts of the body. Often this will follow a general pattern. In prostate cancer, metastatic disease will typically extend to the regional lymph nodes, and then the bones of the hip or lower back. Eventually, the disease will threaten the life of the host.

Not too long ago, the diagnosis of cancer was seen as equivelent to a sentence of death. But recent decades have seen tremendous advancement in cancer treatment. Today, some cancers, such as skin cancer or Hodgkin's disease, are seldom fatal if treated in a timely fashion. Some remain very dangerous. But rarely is a cancer untreatable. There are millions alive today who have conquered their cancer. And progress continues. Some believe

that we are even now on the verge of deciphering
the origins of cancer within the body.

The Cause of Cancer

Much about the manner in which cancer
begins and proliferates remains mysterious. One
thing is clear: damage to a critical portion of the
cell's genetic code must occur for the cell to
become cancerous. The cancer cell then replicates
itself by division, and produces new generations
of altered cells, bearing the genetic errors that
produce cancer.

The genetic code for human beings is about
three billion "letters" long, and is reproduced in
every cell in the body. This code is broken up
among hundreds of thousands of genes. Damaged
cancer-causing genes have been given the name
oncogenes, a combination of the Greek root *onco,*
meaning "tumor," and gene. The discovery of oncogenes in the 1970s opened up new vistas of
scientific exploration into cancer and its causes.

Not every gene has the potential to become an
oncogene. Those genes that can by random error
be transformed into cancer-causing genes are
called *proto-oncogenes.* They are typically involved
in the signaling mechanisms that control cellular
growth and differentiation. Researchers have isolated dozens of these proto-oncogenes. It has been
found that some oncogenes, such as an oncogene
in bladder cancer, differ from the normal, func-

tioning genes by only a single "letter" in the genetic code.

There are several different means under investigation by which proto-oncogenes may become cancer genes. These include:

- Mutations caused by some outside agent, such as radiation or contact with a carcinogen, such as cigarette smoke.

- Gene amplification, which is the production of too many copies of the same gene.

- Chromosomal translocation, or the rearrangement of genes.

Several oncogenes may be involved in the development of a particular kind of cancer. It has been estimated that ten to fifteen genetic changes may be required to develop lung cancer. Research is underway to identify those oncogenes involved in the development of prostate cancer as well. Researchers hope that once the mechanisms that produce prostate cancer are known, they can be counteracted on a molecular level.

The emergence of a cancer cell somewhere in the body does not mean that cancer will persist and proliferate. Many cancers are destroyed by the immune system before a serious malignancy can develop. Why the immune system successfully counteracts the development of these abnormal cells in some instances and fails in others is a matter of speculation. Some believe the immune system must be weakened or altered before an early cancer can advance. This has led to a new avenue of cancer research which seeks to fortify the immune system, called immunotherapy. The recent discovery of the tumor suppressor gene has also become the focus of much attention. When functioning properly, the tumor suppressor gene will sense abnormal cell growth, and activate, causing the offending cells to die. Failure of this gene may also be involved in the inability of the body to control malignant growth.

Reducing Your Risk of Prostate Cancer

These breakthroughs have expanded our knowledge of the origin and progression of cancer, and led to many new fields of research. In the future, this research may lead to the eradication of cancer in all its forms.

But what does this information mean to us today? Since the roots of cancer are genetic, we know that our own genetic make-up may put us at increased risk. Statistics on the incidence of prostate cancer bear this out (*see Fig. 2*). Although random autopsies have shown that as many as 30% of men over 50 will have prostate cancer, only about 1% of these men will be diagnosed or ever experience symptoms of their disease. Clearly, the disease remains latent in most, but those with a family history of cancer are at increased risk. They will be more likely to be among those men in whom the disease advances to the point where it becomes a health problem. Black Americans are also at greater risk — they

Prostate Cancer: The Genetic Link

No family history of cancer .... 1 in 9 (11.2%)

Family history of cancer other than prostate .... 2 in 9 (18.9%)

Both parents with cancer other than prostate .... 2 in 5 (42.6%)

Father had prostate cancer, mother other cancer .... 1 in 2 (53.1%)

Father and uncle(s) with prostate cancer .... 3 in 5 (61.7%)

Grandfather, father and uncle(s) had prostate cancer .... 4 in 5 (86.3%)

Fig. 2: Courtesy of Patient Advocates For Advanced Cancer Treatment (PAACT).

are twice as likely to get prostate cancer as whites. Incidence of the disease in the U.S. is lowest among Asian Americans. Someday gene analysis may identify those who possess the oncogenes that lead to cancer. Until then, those who are at greater risk are advised to take precautions. It is vital to get a regular medical checkup that includes a prostate exam, and if any symptoms of prostate cancer develop, see a doctor immediately.

Other precautions can be taken as well. These precautions are not only preventative, but also apply to anyone who presently has prostate cancer, or wishes to avoid a recurrence of the disease (for further information on self-help methods, *see Chapter 9: Fitness, Diet, and Nutrition*).

• *Avoid known carcinogens.* Those factors in our environment that increase our likelihood of acquiring cancer are known as carcinogens (cancer-causing agents), and should be avoided. Smoking is a known carcinogen, closely associated with lung cancer and bladder cancer. Excessive exposure to sunlight puts us at risk for acquiring skin cancer. Radiation too in a variety of forms is known to promote cancer. Alcohol has been shown to stimulate the growth of cancer. Although none of these is clearly associated with prostate cancer, it is in our general interest to eliminate them from our lives as best we can.

Do not be overly concerned with the latest "carcinogen-of-the-month," the most recent food or chemical that appears in the media as a link to cancer. Most of these are based on limited data, and are frequently contradicted by later studies.

• *Maintain a balanced, nutritional diet.* Although no specific foods have been convincingly identified as carcinogenic, the National Cancer Institute has published guidelines that may be of benefit in resisting cancer. A high-fiber, low-fat diet with at least the minimum recommended dietary allowances (RDAs) for vitamins and minerals is advised.

High fat intake has been statistically associated with an increased risk of prostate cancer. Thus, it is best to limit consumption of such sources of dietary fat as beef, milk products, pork, and eggs.

• *Reduce stress.* Stress can weaken the immune system, essential in fighting off the disease.

• *Maintain good health.* This includes not only watching your diet, but also regular, moderate exercise and plenty of sleep. A stronger body is better able to resist the introduction or spread of disease.

• *Keep a positive attitude.* We now know that an individual's emotions and attitude can impact his body's response to disease. A positive attitude can bolster the immune system as it wages war against the cancer.

Chapter 5

CONDITIONS OF THE PROSTATE

"Just the facts, ma'am."

Sergeant Friday

The Prostate and Surrounding Organs

The prostate is a walnut-size gland at the base of the bladder, surrounding an inch-long segment of the urethra, the passageway through which urine passes out of the body. A male sex organ, the primary function of the prostate is to manufacture the fluid in semen needed for the transport and nourishment of sperm at ejaculation.

There are a number of surrounding organs intimately associated with the prostate and its functions (*see Fig. 3*). The seminal vesicles are two sac-like structures that contain a nutrient fluid for the spermatozoa and are situated behind the

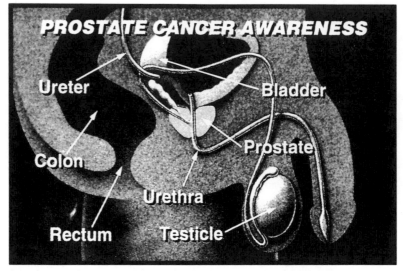

Figure 3: The prostate and surrounding organs. This illustration shows the entire male genitourinary tract, with specific reference to the prostate and those organs with which it is in close relationship.

bladder. They connect to the prostatic urethra by way of the ejaculatory ducts. The external urethral sphincter is a band of muscle directly below the prostate, and functions to shut off the flow of urine. Sperm produced in the testicles are carried up to the prostate by way of paired muscular cords known as the vas deferens. It is these cords that are surgically severed in a vasectomy.

Prostate Anatomy

The first detailed description of the prostate's anatomy, made in 1912, divided the gland into five separate lobes. More recently, a revised anatomy of the prostate has been developed which divides

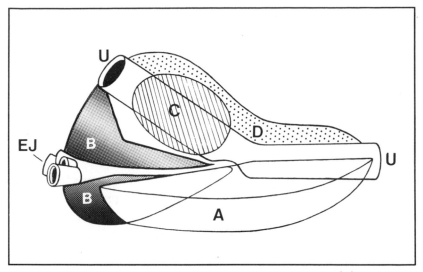

Figure 4: McNeal's zonal anatomy of the prostate, showing the (A) peripheral, (B) central, and (C) transitional zones, as well as the (U) urethra, (EJ) ejaculatory ducts and (D) anterior fibromuscular stroma.

the prostate into several zones, based on cellular variations in the tissue of the prostate gland (*see Fig. 4*).

This zonal anatomy, developed by McNeal, has distinguished three basic zones of glandular tissue in the prostate, the central, transitional and peripheral zones. There is also a nonglandular region known as the anterior fibromuscular stroma. The central zone surrounds the ejaculatory ducts and makes up approximately 25% of the prostate. It is rarely the site of origin of prostate cancer —– no more than 5% to 10% of diagnosed cases. The capsular covering that surrounds the prostate gland is weakest at the point where the seminal vesicles and the vas deferens cords enter the central zone. Under normal conditions, the transitional zone comprises only 5% of the prostate and carcinomas arising in the transitional zone account for about 10% to 20% of prostate cancers. The peripheral zone comprises about 70% of the glandular prostate. About 80% of cancers are believed to originate in the peripheral zone of the prostate.

McNeal's zonal anatomy of the prostate has distinct advantages. The histological variations within the prostate reflect sound waves differently, often allowing identification of the prostate's zones with a transrectal ultrasound test. Cancerous tumors within particular zones of the prostate will also often be distinguishable with ultrasound. This has prognostic value to the physician, since the characteristics of tumors located in particular zones often fall into certain basic categories. Carcinomas of the central or transitional zone typically exhibit a low level of malignancy. On the other hand, peripheral zone carcinomas tend to have a worse prognosis.

Common Prostate Problems

A variety of prostate problems are common in men over 50. The symptoms of these conditions are often similar or overlap. The presence of any of these symptoms frequently cause men to prematurely conclude they have prostate cancer. In fact, symptoms of a prostate disorder are far more likely to be the consequence of a benign condition, such as one of the following:

Acute Prostatitis

A condition that can afflict men of any age, it is a bacterial infection that has spread to the prostate from elsewhere in the body. Symptoms include a high fever, flu-like aches and pains, and pain in the lower back or between the legs. Because this condition causes significant swelling of the prostate, the individual with acute prostatitis may experience painful or difficult urination. Usually, this condition can be treated successfully with antibiotics and bed rest.

Chronic Prostatitis

A recurring inflammation or infection of the prostate. The condition is typically milder than acute prostatitis, and is seldom accompanied by a fever. When bacteria are present in the prostate, the cause can usually be traced to a lingering infection from an earlier case of acute prostatitis. When so diagnosed, antibiotics are prescribed. Sometimes no bacteria can be found associated with the inflammation of the prostate. In these cases, inflammation is attributed to an enlargement of the prostate caused by an excess of secreted fluids within the gland. Although symptoms may persist for some time, the condition will usually clear up of its own accord.

Prostatodynia

Contrary to its name, this rare medical condition does not actually originate in the prostate, but is usually an inflammation located in the pelvic bones or associated muscle tissues. Because it produces similar symptoms ---- such as pain in the area of the prostate, between the legs ---- it is sometimes misdiagnosed as prostatitis. When properly diagnosed, prostatodynia is usually treated with muscle relaxants and anti-inflammatory agents.

Benign Prostatic Hypertrophy (BPH)

Also called benign prostatic hyperplasia, this condition is an enlargement of the prostate that begins with most men around the age of 50. It is caused by the growth of benign (non-cancerous) tumors originating in the transition zone at the core of the prostate. Although poorly understood, BPH is clearly related to hormonal changes that occur with aging.

Although many men with BPH never experience significant problems as a result of the condition, given sufficient time, symptoms will begin to manifest themselves. As the prostate gland grows larger, the BPH tissue will begin to constrict the prostatic urethra. Eventually, this will result in symptoms such as difficulty in urination, decreased or interrupted flow, and the urge to urinate frequently.

When it reaches an advanced stage, BPH can have severe and even life-threatening effects. As BPH worsens, residual urine may be left in the bladder, leading to recurrent bladder infections, kidney damage, overflow incontinence, or the inability to urinate. At this point, it is essential that the condition be treated.

There are a variety of medications a doctor can prescribe to alleviate the symptoms of BPH, such as alpha adrenergic blockers, like Hytrin, and agents that interfere with the production of testosterone, such as the new drug, Proscar. None are to date curative. As the condition progresses, surgery may become the only alternative. The most common surgical approach to BPH is called a transurethral resection of the prostate (TURP), a procedure which involves the use of a surgical instrument called a resectoscope to trim BPH tissue from the prostate gland from within the prostatic urethra. If the prostate is extremely enlarged, an open surgical procedure known as a simple prostatectomy may be indicated (*see Treatment Options, p. 73*).

Prostate cancer may exist in combination with benign conditions, such as BPH. Since the symptoms of prostate cancer (*see chart on next page*) resemble or are in some cases identical with symptoms for benign conditions, appropriate diagnostic tests must be performed to make an accurate diagnosis.

Symptoms of Prostate Cancer

* Blood in urine (hematuria).

* Pain or difficulty urinating.

* Increased frequency of urination, often at night (nocturia).

* Increased voiding urgency.

* Hesitant or intermittent urinary flow.

* Inability to urinate.

* Pain or discomfort in area of prostate.

Unusual and unexplained weight loss.

Continual pain in bones of lower back, hips or pelvis.

Figure 5. Those symptoms marked with an * may be due to benign conditions of the prostate, entirely unrelated to prostate cancer.

Cancer of the Prostate

Like benign prostatic hypertrophy (BPH), carcinoma of the prostate causes an enlargement of the prostate gland, and produces symptoms of urinary obstruction. Unlike BPH, prostate cancer typically fails to produce any symptoms during the early stages of its development. This is because these two conditions characteristically arise in two different sites within the prostate (*see Fig. 6*). BPH grows within the transitional zone, near the core of the prostate, and for this reason, its expansion will begin to constrict the urethra relatively early in its development. Prostate cancer

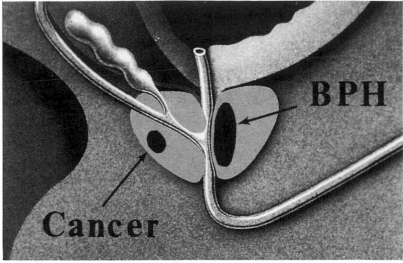

Figure 6. A prostate gland showing BPH and cancer. BPH usually begins near the core, while in most cases prostate cancer arises near the boundary of the gland.

typically originates in the periphery of the gland, near the boundary of the prostate known as the prostatic capsule. As a consequence, the cancerous tumor will often penetrate the capsule of the prostate and spread to other areas of the body, long before it has penetrated far enough inward toward the center of the prostate to put pressure of the prostatic urethra and produce symptoms. Because no symptoms may appear for months or years while this disease progresses, early prostate cancer has been labeled the "silent disease." In fact, the earliest indication of the disease may be pain in the lower back, hips or pelvis, indicating spread of cancer to the bones. At that point, the disease is considered incurable. This highlights the importance of annual physical examinations for the early detection of the often surreptitious disease known as prostate cancer.

Chapter 6

DIAGNOSIS AND STAGING OF PROSTATE CANCER

*If we could first know where we are and whither
we are tending, we could better judge what to do
and how to do it.*

Abraham Lincoln

Diagnosis

New techniques have led to significant progress in the early detection of prostate cancer in recent years. Also, an increased awareness of the problem has given men greater incentive to include an examination of the prostate as part of their annual physicals. As a consequence, a greater number of men are being diagnosed with prostate cancer while the disease is still at an early stage and most treatable.

Even so, among all men diagnosed with prostate cancer, whether due to routine physical examination or after the appearance of symptoms, studies indicate that over half will be found to have disease that has spread beyond the prostate. And among those men who wait until symptoms present themselves, the vast majority will have late stage prostate cancer, or disease that is no longer confined to the prostate. These facts are particularly compelling since, although there are effective means of treating the disease, late stage prostate cancer is presently considered incurable.

My own case was an exception. The tumor in my prostate started much closer to the prostatic urethra than in most men. As a result, I was very fortunate to have symptoms of the disease while the cancer remained confined to the prostate. But most will not be so lucky. If you have not yet been diagnosed with prostate cancer and are at risk (that is, if you are male and over 40!), I strongly urge you to take advantage of the methods of early detection presently available.

Below are the techniques presently in use for the early detection and diagnosis of prostate cancer:

Digital Rectal Examination (DRE)

This technique has been in use for decades and remains the most common method for detecting the presence of prostate cancer. To examine the prostate, a physician inserts a lubricated, gloved finger into the patient's rectum to feel the size and shape of the prostate through the rectum wall. An enlarged prostate may indicate cancer, but is more commonly the result of a benign condition, particularly BPH. Areas on the surface of the prostate that feel nodular, lumpy or harder than surrounding tissues may indicate the presence of a cancer tumor. In cases of an enlarged or irregular prostate, a biopsy should be performed, and the tissue examined microscopically for cancer. Further tests may also be in order.

With the DRE, only the posterior portion of the prostate can be palpated. Those tumors located elsewhere, or tumors that are small or diffuse, will often be undetectable by DRE. Also, only about 20% of those with a positive DRE (that is, some abnormality was found during the examination) will actually have prostate cancer. Nonetheless, at this time, many doctors consider it the most effective screening test for prostate cancer.

The procedure can be performed in under a minute with little discomfort to the patient. Many men feel unnecessarily squeamish about this test, but given the high incidence of prostate cancer, it should be included in annual physical exams for any man over 40.

Prostate Specific Antigen (PSA) test

A blood test that measures the level of prostate specific antigen (PSA) present in the body. PSA is a protein produced exclusively within the prostate, and typically present only in minute quantities in the blood stream. Because cancerous cells readily leak PSA into the surrounding body tissue, an elevated PSA is a possible indicator of the presence of prostate cancer. Prostate enlargement due to benign prostatic hypertrophy (BPH) can also cause an increase in PSA levels. The normal range for PSA is between 0 and 4.0 ng/ml (nanograms per millileter), although this may vary based on the age of a patient. Serum PSA levels between 4.0 and 10.0 ng/ml may be due to prostate cancer, BPH, or some other condition. In two thirds of the cases, if the serum PSA level is above 10.0 ng/ml, the patient has prostate cancer, usually with disease no longer confined to the prostate. However, there are cases where the PSA level can get as high as 100 ng/ml with no sign of cancer. For those with advanced metastatic disease, the PSA value may rise into the hundreds.

The PSA blood test is a recent advance in the detection of prostate cancer, and is usually able to detect carcinoma of the prostate at an earlier stage than the DRE. Due to its greater sensitivity, the PSA test has almost entirely replaced the older PAP (prostatic acid phosphatase) blood test in general use. Furthermore, the PSA test has proved twice as accurate as the DRE — 40% of cases showing elevated PSA levels will prove to have prostate cancer.

Nonetheless, the serum PSA test has not escaped criticism. The test is not foolproof. Occasionally, prostate cancer will not produce an elevated PSA level. And when the PSA level is less than 10 ng/ml, false positive results are very high, prompting many physicians to question the value of the PSA test as a screening test for cancer. Recent studies, however, indicate that the vast majority of prostate cancers identified with PSA testing are more virulent forms, and will eventually pose a health risk. PSA testing is best used in combination with the DRE, which results in an improved detection rate and fewer false positive results.

Transrectal Ultrasonography of the Prostate (TRUS)

This is the procedure known to the layman as ultrasound. A small instrument is inserted into the rectum which produces sound waves that reflect off the prostate, producing an image. Ultrasonography has proven ineffective when used as the primary tool for early detection of prostate cancer, and leads to a very high number of unnecessary biopsies. However, prostate tumors frequently reflect sound waves differently than surrounding tissues. As a follow-up test used when DRE and/or PSA tests yeild suspicious results, transrectal ultrasound can provide useful information for the identification of prostate abnormalities. At the time of the ultrasound examination, the physician will often perform a needle biopsy, removing a tissue sample from any suspicious looking area. The development of ultrasound-guided biopsy has much improved the accuracy of biopsy results, often locating cancerous tumors in the prostate that were missed by DRE guided biopsy.

Biopsy

A biopsy is the removal of a sample of tissue from a suspicious area of the prostate for examination by a pathologist. This procedure is absolutely necessary to verify the presence of cancer, and should be undertaken prior to any treatment for prostate cancer. Pathological examination of the biopsy sample also provides a wealth of information concerning the characteristics of the cancer.

A biopsy may be taken in a number of ways. The traditional method involves the use of a large, hollow needle with which a core or plug of prostate tissue, about a millimeter in diameter, may be taken. The needle may be guided by the finger of the physician during rectal examination, or with the use of ultrasound, which provides the doctor with an interior view of the prostate as the sample is taken from the suspected area. An alternate method, known as "needle aspiration of the prostate" involves a "skinny needle," and uses a syringe to draw a tiny amount of prostate material into the end of the needle. This method has the advantage of being less uncomfortable than the core sample biopsy, but requires greater expertise both in sampling and in pathological examination of the biopsy tissue.

At this point, there does not seem to be a consensus in the medical community concerning the proper role of these tests in early detection of prostate cancer. Some physicians feel that the PSA test should be part of every man's regular physical examination, once he reaches age 50. Others feel that PSA and ultrasound tests put unnecessary stress and financial burden upon their patients due to the inappropriately high number of false positive results (cases where the test indicates prostate cancer when no cancer exists). There is also concern that latent or insignificant cancers may be discovered ---- tumors that would never pose a threat to the patient during his lifetime --- and treated unnecessarily.

At present, the best advice seems to be to include both a digital rectal exam (DRE) and PSA blood test in your annual physical after age 40. The PSA blood test will not greatly increase the cost of your yearly examination ---- it usually runs about $50. If both the DRE and PSA test are positive, or if the PSA level jumps dramatically from one year to the next, follow up with an ultrasound guided biopsy.

Let the medical community worry about what is appropriate as a screening method for the general public. As an individual, it is in your best interests to use the available early detection techniques. Catching the disease early can dramatically improve your chances of successful treatment.

Evaluation and Staging

Once the presence of prostate cancer has been positively identified, the physician will base his prognosis and recommended treatment options upon two factors: an evaluation of the nature of the malignancy, and a determination of the stage, or extent, of the cancer.

An evaluation of the nature of the malignancy will aid in predicting how rapidly and aggressively the cancer will grow and spread. This evaluation is made by the pathologist upon microscopic examination and analysis of cancer cells in the biopsy sample. First, the cancer cells are graded by degree of differentiation (that is, the degree to which they resemble normal, healthy cells of the prostate). There are several grading systems, but the most commonly used is known as the Gleason grading system (*see Fig. 7*). This system has defined five glandular patterns of cancerous cell tissue under low magnification, from completely differentiated to completely undifferentiated. Some tumors will possess more than one cellular pattern, and so both the primary and secondary patterns are graded. The two grades are combined to get a Gleason score, ranging from 2 (1 + 1) to 10 (5 + 5), with most cancers falling somewhere in between. Gleason scores at the low and high ends of the scale ---- 2 to 4 and 8 to 10 respectively ---- have been shown to effectively predict the behavior of a tumor. Those graded in the low range are

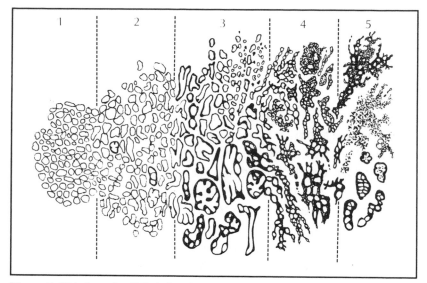

Figure 7. This is a simplified drawing of the Gleason grading system, showing the five distinct grades of cancerous tissue, as seen under low magnification. The two most common cell patterns seen in a tissue sample are added together to generate a Gleason score.

significantly less likely to grow rapidly and spread, whereas a high score indicates that the cancer is aggressive, and is likely to expand and metastisize without treatment.

Another test sometimes performed by the pathologist uses a technique called flow cytometry to analyze the nuclear DNA content, or "DNA ploidy," of cancer cells. Aneuploid cancers generally have a worse prognosis than diploid cancers, and if left untreated are more likely to progress rapidly. Localized aneuploid tumors should be considered strong candidates for surgery, regardless of stage. The predictive value of flow cytometry ploidy is significantly enhanced when correlated with the patient's Gleason score.

The Stages

Decades of studies have led to the present classification of prostate cancer into four distinct stages: A, B, C, and D. There are substages for each stage of prostate cancer as well. The stage of prostate cancer is based on such factors as the size or volume of disease, Gleason grade, and spread of disease beyond the prostate or to other sites in the body, such as the seminal vesicles, pelvic lymph nodes, or more distant lungs or bones.

To determine the stage of disease, the physician must take into account information gained during diagnosis and pathological analysis. Also, additional tests will typically be required to ensure an accurate determination of the stage of cancer. *Accurate staging of the disease is crucial to developing an appropriate treatment plan.*

There are a wide variety of staging tests, each possessing unique capabilities and serving a specific function in the staging process. Some tests are used to visualize the internal structures of the body, such as the CT scan, MRI, or ultrasound. Others are used to identify the presence of cancer in various parts of the body, such as the chest x-ray or bone scan. Blood tests may be used to give a general indication of the extensiveness of the disease, such as the PSA and PAP tests. These tests may be used for preliminary staging and for subsequent staging to track changes in a patient's illness or evaluate the effectiveness of treatment.

A determination of stage based on these clinical tests, without direct examination of the tumor or cancer cells, is known as "clinical staging." Although the tests used in staging are always undergoing improvement and refinement, clinical staging is not foolproof. Staging tests provide valuable information to the physician, but unavoidable errors in assessing the stage still do occur. "Surgical staging" provides more precise and verifiable data on the extent of the disease. It is accomplished by means of biopsy or surgical exploration. Because prostate cancer tends to spread to the pelvic lymph nodes once it metastisizes, a surgical technique called a lymphadenectomy is sometimes performed to sample the lymph nodes for verification of the spread of disease. "Pathological staging" refers to the determination of the stage of disease based on direct microscopic examination of biopsies and surgical specimens. It is the most precise means of determining the extent of disease. For a description of the various staging tests and their use, see *Appendix D: Diagnostic and Staging Tests*.

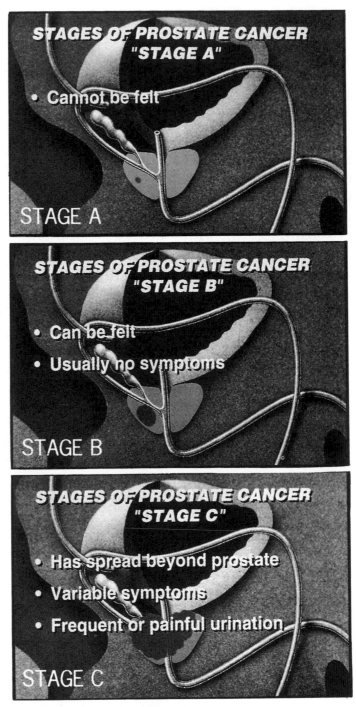

Illustrations courtesy of TAP Pharmaceuticals, Inc.

Description of Stages

STAGE A: These are cancers confined to the prostate that cannot be felt during rectal examination, and produce no symptoms. Usually, stage A tumors are found by accident during routine examination of tissue removed during surgery for benign prostatic hypertrophy (BPH). As many as 10% of men who undergo transurethral resection of the prostate (TURP) for BPH are discovered to have unsuspected prostate cancer. On rare occasions, stage A cancers are discovered incidentally using ultrasound. This stage is further divided into two substages.

- STAGE A1: Although there is some variance in definitions of this sub-stage, typically a focalized tumor (spherical and possessing a distinct boundary between the tumor and surrounding tissue) that has a Gleason score of 5 or less, and comprises 5% or less of the surgical specimen.

- STAGE A2: Typically a diffuse tumor, which exhibits poor differentiation (Gleason score greater than 5), or one that makes up over 5% of the removed specimen of prostate tissue.

STAGE B: The tumor can be felt by rectal examination, but is still confined to the prostate gland.

- STAGE B1: The tumor is less than 2 centimeters in diameter and confined to one lobe of the prostate.

- STAGE B2: The cancer is 2 centimeters or more in diameter, or involves both sides of the prostate gland.

STAGE C: Cancer that has extended through the prostatic capsule, and is no longer confined to the prostate. Stage C cancers often involve most or all of the prostate gland, and the entire prostate may feel hard upon rectal examination. Those cancers which have spread to the seminal vesicles are also considered stage C carcinomas. Often symptoms of the disease will begin to appear at this stage of the disease, such as difficulty urinating.

STAGE D: The prostate cancer has spread beyond the prostate and its immediate surroundings.

- STAGE D1: Prostate cancer has invaded the regional lymph nodes.

- STAGE D2: Prostate cancer has spread to distant sites in the body. Metastatic disease will usually spread to nearby bones, but may also involve the liver, lungs or other tissues.

Chapter 7

TREATMENT OPTIONS

"We are born to inquire into truth."

Michel De Montaigne

Overview

Presently, treatment alternatives for prostate cancer are classified as "curative" or "palliative." Those patients who have early stage prostate cancer (stages A and B) are candidates for curative treatments. Traditionally, the treatment options for such patients have been limited to the surgical procedure known as a radical prostatectomy, and radiation therapy, such as is used with many other forms of cancer. Both have seen significant advances in recent years. But within the last decade, a number of new techniques have been developed for the treatment of early stage prostate cancer. While most remain investigational, these recent developments have given men a wider range of alternatives than ever before.

Those with late stage disease, or disease that has spread beyond the prostate gland, are generally considered incurable using presently available techniques. Many of those who read this book may fall into this category — perhaps you are one of them. But if you have late stage prostate cancer, don't give up hope simply because the medical community presently considers your condition incurable. Prostate cancer is a very unpredictable disease: many men even with metastatic disease have lived for a decade or more with little or no progression of the cancer. Many eventually die of natural causes. And there are even the rare instances of spontaneous remission.

More importantly, there are several treatment options that remain for those patients with late stage prostate cancer which can be successfully used to slow or halt progression of the disease and to alleviate symptoms.

Experimentation into the efficacy of a wide array of drugs is also underway, any one of which may be key to a new or improved form of treatment for prostate cancer. And as research continues into the the causal foundations of cancer, some day in the not too distant future a cure for any and all stages of prostate cancer may be found.

Current Treatments

Following are general descriptions of currently available forms of treatment. To find more information on these forms of therapy, *see Appendix A: Where to Get Help.*

Radical Prostatectomy

Unlike the "simple" prostatectomy, performed in severe cases of BPH (benign prostatic hypertrophy) to remove excess tissue, this procedure involves the total removal of the prostate gland, as well as the seminal vesicles and a certain amount of surrounding tissue. For this reason, it is also known as a "total" prostatectomy. It is intended as a curative treatment, and thus usually only patients with early stage prostate cancer are candidates for the operation. There are two forms of the operation, based on whether a "retropubic" or "perineal" surgical approach is used. Both have advantages and disadvantages.

The *radical retropubic prostatectomy* is the most common form of the operation. The most significant advantage of this approach is that it allows for the examination of pelvic lymph nodes, to which cancer typically spreads after it leaves the prostate. Although diagnostic tests for identifying cancer in the lymph nodes have improved dramatically over the past several years, only removal and examination of the lymph nodes can verify the presence or absence of cancer. This is important since involvement of the lymph nodes would mean the patient is no longer a candidate for cure using a radical prostatectomy. And once the physician is alerted that the patient has late stage disease, an appropriate alternative treatment can be initiated.

The patient is first anesthetized, and a long vertical incision is made in the lower abdomen, from the navel to the pubic bone. Once the incision is made, the surgeon will usually remove for examination some of the pelvic lymph nodes. The removed lymph nodes are immediately sent to the pathologist for "frozen section" analysis, a quick procedure which takes about 20 minutes. The pathologist sends the results of the analysis back to the surgeon.

If cancer is found in the lymph nodes, the surgeon must decide if he should continue or abort the operation. Most urologists feel that there is little rationale for putting the patient through the operation with no chance of cure. However, some feel that if there is only minor involvement of the lymph nodes, removal of the primary tumor, located in the prostate, may be of advantage for the patient both in reducing symptoms of the disease and extending the patient's life.

If no cancer is found by the pathologist, the operation can proceed. Access to the prostate is gained by going behind the pubic bone (hence the name "retropubic"). The removal of the prostate is begun just above the external urethral sphincter. The prostatic urethra is divided, and the prostate is surgically removed, along with the seminal vesicles behind the bladder. The bladder neck is cut and the prostate is removed in its entirety. Then the bladder neck is pulled downwards and stitched to the severed end of the urethra. During this final phase of the operation, a Foley catheter is inserted into the penis, and up into the bladder to control drainage of urine. The abdominal incision is stitched up and the operation is over.

Although to the layman, the prostate seems a small organ, and thus should require relatively minor surgery to remove, this procedure is actually quite formidable. It may take up to four hours to perform, and because there are numerous blood vessels in the area of the prostate, the operation often entails considerable loss of blood. Post-operative care involves a hospital stay sometimes as long as 10 days to two weeks, after which the patient can go home. The catheter remains in place for about three weeks, and is removed on a return visit to the doctor's office.

The *radical perineal prostatectomy* approaches the prostate through the perineum, the area between the scrotum and the anus. The principle advantage of this approach is that the post-operative recovery is much easier on the patient. However, this procedure does not allow for the dissection and examination of regional lymph nodes. As a consequence, most urologists reserve this technique for those with small, localized tumors, in which the likelihood of cancerous lymph nodes is very small. Some surgeons who use the perineal approach first perform an exploratory lymphadenectomy. After a few days, if the pathologist's report indicates that the lymph nodes are clear of cancer, the surgeon performs the prostatectomy.

The risks and complications associated with a radical prostatectomy are considerable. There is a mortality rate of 1%-2% for those who undergo the operation. Consequently, candidates for the operation are typically limited to men in good health and under the age of 70. The most serious and distressing complications of this operation are urinary incontinence and erectile dysfunction. The skill of the surgeon can significantly reduce the long-term complications of this procedure.

Loss of bladder control ranges from mild incontinence (such as stress incontinence), which may endure for a period of several days to many months following the operation, to severe incontinence, due to permanent damage done to the urethral sphincter. Severe incontinence occurs in about 5% of patients, but even in these cases, exercises, medications or the surgical placement of an artificial sphincter may be used to restore urinary control to the patient (*see Coping with Complications, p. 163*).

Loss of sexual function is very common, since two nerve bundles closely associated with erection are located just outside the top portion of the prostate gland. A new technique, pioneered by Dr. James Walsh at Johns Hopkins, preserves one

or both of these nerves during the radical prostatectomy. In theory, this nerve-sparing technique allows a majority of patients to retain
sexual function. However, because the technique
requires shaving close to the side margins of the
prostate, it is often reserved for patients whose
cancer is most likely to be contained within the
capsule of the prostate. Drugs such as papaverine
can be used to treat impotence resulting from the
operation, and if necessary, a penile prosthesis may
be employed (*see Coping with Complications, p. 163*).

Radiation Therapy

Since the 1950s, external radiation therapy has
been a common technique used for the treatment
of many kinds of cancers. It is a standard treatment
for prostate cancer that is clinically confined to
the prostate and surrounding tissues (stages A, B,
and C). On rare occasions, it is recommended for
those patients with stage D1 disease, prostate
cancer that has spread to the pelvic lymph nodes.
Radiation therapy is also used as an adjuvant
therapy in those cases where residual cancer is
found following a radical prostatectomy. High
energy X-rays are targeted upon the region of the
prostate to kill or incapacitate any cancer cells
in the area. Although healthy tissues are also
damaged, normal cells are better able to recover
and survive the radiation. Treatment is administered four to five times a week for a period of six
or seven weeks. Each treatment takes about
three minutes. The machines used to administer

external beam radiation are the Cobalt 60 unit, the linear accelerator, and the betatron. Cobalt units have been in use the longest and are still used in many institutions, but because they employ a lower voltage, there is more scatter of radiation with these machines. Consequently, they are significantly more likely to produce deleterious side effects, and should be avoided.

As with radical prostatectomy, there are many possible complications of external radiation therapy. Among the side effects that occur during the course of treatment are fatigue, nausea, diarrhea, bowel irritation and painful urination. The majority of these symptoms will disappear after treatment is concluded, but in some cases, damage to the bladder or, less frequently, to the rectum results in chronic complications. These include bladder inflammation and the need to urinate frequently (cystitis) in about 10% of patients, or intermittent periods of diarrhea that may continue for years afterwards. Severe rectal injury is rare. Although most men retain potency after the conclusion of radiation therapy, as many as half of the men who undergo this treatment will eventually develop erectile dysfunction. The mechanism which produces this impotence is poorly understood. For those men who are no longer able to achieve erection, a penile implant may be necessary to restore sexual function (*see Coping with Complications, p. 163*).

The skill of the radiotherapist administering treatments can significantly reduce the likelihood of these complications. Preparation for radiation therapy is a precise and complex process, involving the exact determination of the region to receive treatment and the appropriate dose of radiation.

There is much disagreement concerning whether radiation therapy is as effective as radical prostatectomy for curing prostate cancer. Statistical analyses, although usually favoring radical prostatectomy, shows the results of the two treatments are roughly comparable in outcome up to 10 years after treatment. However, biopsies performed on patients who have undergone radiation therapy indicate that half or more of these men have residual cancer of the prostate. One present theory suggests that radiation therapy may in most cases only halt the progression of the disease for a number of years, after which it will recur. Many radiotherapists argue that this is only the case if the radiation beam is imprecisely directed during treatment. The use of a new three-dimensional computerized imaging technique has much improved the accuracy of external radiation of the prostate. Early results from this technique, also known as "conformal therapy," have been very good, thus corroborating the position of the radiotherapists. In one study, only 15% of patients biopsied after 3-D radiation therapy showed residual cancer. In addition, side effects of the treatment are also less common than with the traditional application of radiation therapy. Unfortunately, this new technique is not widely available at this time.

Transurethral Resection of the Prostate (TURP)

This is an operation typically used to treat symptoms of urinary obstruction. Most often, it is used to treat the benign condition referred to as BPH (*see p. 52*), but may also be used to relieve obstruction produced by prostate cancer. The procedure involves the insertion of a specialized surgical instrument called a resectoscope into the penis and up the urethra to the interior of the prostate. Tissue is carefully cut away from the walls of the prostatic urethra with an electrical wire, until the passage permits the unobstructed flow of urine from the bladder. Afterwards a Foley catheter is introduced into the bladder to control the drainage of urine, and must remain in place for several days following the surgery.

Because no incision is made, the patient will experience minimal discomfort, and is only hospitalized for a brief period following the procedure. However, the TURP is a very difficult procedure. Not only is there considerable risk of blood loss during the surgery, but there is the danger of injury to the bladder neck and urethral sphincter, which can lead to bladder neck contracture or urinary incontinence. To avoid these complications, the urologist performing the operation must be expert in this form of surgery.

It is not uncommon for prostate cancer to be initially discovered following the examination of tissue removed during the TURP. These are typically stage A carcinomas of the prostate. Occasionally, repeat TURPs are performed for staging purposes, to determine if there is any residual cancer remaining in the prostate.

Brachytherapy

Also called "interstitial implantation therapy," this treatment involves the implantation of radioactive seeds into the prostate. A relatively common investigational technique since its development in the early 1970s, due to recent improvements in the procedure, brachytherapy is growing in popularity. The earliest form of the seed implantation procedure required major abdominal surgery. After performing a pelvic lymph node dissection, radioactive Iodine-125 seeds contained in the tips of needles were manually implanted into the prostate in rows one centimeter apart. The procedure fell out of favor because seed placement was less than ideal. More recently, a non-invasive technique has been developed for placing the radioactive seeds in the prostate without resorting to open surgery. Hollow needles used to dispense the radioactive seeds are inserted through the perineum — the area between the scrotum and anus — implementing a positioned template to guide placement. A further refinement of the procedure, gaining widespread acceptance over the past few years, employs realtime imaging — usually with the use of transrectal ultrasound, but occasionally using CT scanning or fluoroscopy — to ensure precise placement of the seeds in the prostate. A few years ago this technique using ultrasound guidance was available in only a few states. Low complication rates and promising clinical results have contributed to its widening availability.

A number of radioactive sources have been used for interstitial implantation. The most commonly used permanent implants are radioactive seeds using encapsulated Iodine-125 and the newly available Palladium-103. Palladium-103 has a significantly shorter half-life (that is, the period of time until the source's output of radiation is halved) and greater initial radioactive dose rate than Iodine-125. Thus, in theory it is more likely to be effective against rapidly growing, highly malignant cancers.

Brachytherapy with ultrasound guidance has certain advantages over the traditionally used external beam radiation therapy. Because radiation will damage healthy tissue as well as cancerous tissue, the standard dose of radiation used externally upon the prostate is about 7000 rads, calculated to be the highest dose which is safe and well tolerated by the patient. Radioactive seeds implanted in the prostate deliver radiation only to the prostate itself and not surrounding organs. As a consequence, doses exceeding 12,000 rads can be administered to the area of the prostate using internally implanted radioactive seeds.

This would suggest that brachytherapy should have significantly improved results when compared with treatment using external beam radiation. In the early eighties, the initial studies evaluating the effectiveness of brachytherapy performed without ultrasound guidance were disappointing. There was a higher rate of local recurrence (that is, return of cancer in the prostate after treatment) with brachytherapy than with either the radical prostatectomy or radiation therapy. These poor results were most likely due to inaccurate seed placement, since the procedure was done without ultrasound guidance. Poor placement of radioactive seeds led to "cold" spots within the prostate that do not receive a sufficient dose of radiation.

Although it is still too early for a complete evaluation of ultrasound-guided brachytherapy, the latest findings have been very favorable. Five-year data on patients treated at the Seattle Tumor Institute show disease-free survival rates superior to external radiation and radical prostatectomy in studies with comparable patient samples (*see also Fig. 11 on p. 97*). At the very least, it appears an excellent alternative for older patients or those who wish to avoid the added risks of surgery.

Brachytherapy with guidance offers a new and cost-effective (at about half the price of a radical prostatectomy) means of treating early stage prostate cancer. The operation can be performed in under an hour on an out-patient basis, making it very appealing to those who wish to avoid the risks and hospitalization involved in major surgery. The radioactive seeds remain permanently in place within the prostate. They pose no health threat to the patient, and decay within six to twelve months, at which point they become inert and inactive.

This form of therapy has also resulted in minimal complications. As the radioactive sources decay, some men experience urinary problems involving urgency, frequency, or difficulty urinating. These symptoms generally dissipate by the time the seeds have lost their radioactivity. Incontinence and other serious complications have been very rare, except in those patients who have previously had a transurethral resection of the prostate (TURP). For this reason, this procedure is not recommended for patients who have undergone a TURP procedure. Treatment is also typically restricted to men with prostates less than 60 cc in volume. Most notably, about 90% of men who receive brachytherapy retain their sexual potency, which far exceeds the results obtained with other available curative treatments for prostate cancer.

For more on this procedure, *see Ch. 9: The Healing Seed.*

Cryotherapy

The process of freezing and thawing can disrupt and destroy living tissue. Based on this principle, cryosurgery has been in use for some time, and is effective for the treatment of cervical cancer, and tumors of the head, neck, and skin, as well as other sites.

Early attempts at prostate cryosurgery, undertaken about 30 years ago, resulted in a high level of complications, but the advent of transrectal ultrasound has led to significant improvements in cryosurgical technique for the treatment of prostate cancer. Current therapy involves the freezing of prostate tissue with the use of probes containing liquid nitrogen, inserted through the perineum and into the prostate. Ultrasound is used to guide the placement of the probes, and carefully control the amount of tissue frozen.

The advantages of cryotherapy over radical surgery are substantial. The procedure is performed on an outpatient basis under general anesthesia — no cutting is involved. Prostate tissue destroyed by the procedure is not removed, but is absorbed by the body. Recovery time is brief, and complications thus far have been few. In theory, nerve cells are not permanently damaged by freezing, so cryosurgery may be able to preserve the nerves essential to sexual function. However, in practice, about two-thirds of cryosurgery patients have been rendered impotent by the procedure, although it is unknown how many may regain potency over time.

Preliminary results have been favorable, with about 75% of patients testing negative for cancer on biopsy 3 to 6 months after treatment. However, about half possess PSA values over 0 ng/ml, often rising over time, suggesting residual cancer may remain. It is still far too early to judge the true effectiveness of this investigational treatment as a cure for prostate cancer. Unlike surgery or external radiation, the treatment can be repeated.

Hyperthermia

This is the use of heat to kill cancer cells, and is currently under investigation for several types of cancer tumors, such as tumors of the head, neck, breast, and prostate. Cancer cells do not tolerate heat as well as healthy cells. Hyperthermia also makes the cancer cells more sensitive to radiation or chemotherapy treatment. Thus, it is often used in conjunction with other forms of therapy.

Research into hyperthermia involves several methods for applying heat to the area of the tumor while minimizing damage to surrounding tissue and organs. Laser and microwave-induced hyperthermia is currently under investigation for the treatment of prostate cancer.

Hormonal Therapy

This therapy has become the standard treatment for those whose cancer has extended beyond the prostate, and are thus considered incurable. It has been long-established that the vast majority of prostate cancers are dependent on the male hormone, testosterone. The goal of hormonal therapy is to decrease the production of testosterone in the body, thus inhibiting the growth of the cancer. In most cases, this therapy will also significantly reduce pain and other symptoms of the disease. Patient response to hormonal therapy varies widely. In those that initially respond to treatment, control of the disease may last from several months to many years. A small number with metastatic prostate cancer, possibly as high as 10% of patients, survive for 10 years or more, often with signs of complete disease regression. However, in the great majority of cases, the cancer eventually becomes refractory — or unresponsive — to hormonal manipulation, and the patient will experience a relapse of the disease. It is poorly understood why this occurs, but most likely a form of prostate cancer develops that is "androgen-independent," or unaffected by male hormones. At this point, no form of hormonal therapy is likely to have a significant impact on the disease, and the patient must resort to another form of treatment, such as chemotherapy. There are several available methods used to reduce the production of male hormones by the body. Following are the most common forms of hormonal therapy presently in use.

Bilateral Orchiectomy

This procedure is the surgical removal of the testicles. It is a palliative rather than curative treatment, usually reserved for those with late stage prostate cancer (C or D). The testicles produce about 95% of the body's testosterone, and with their removal, a dramatic impact is often seen. Orchiectomy usually results in a retardation of the growth and spread of the disease. In fact, it is quite common for cancerous tumors to shrink in size after a bilateral orchiectomy is performed. Subjective responses are also striking in the majority of patients, with significant reduction of pain and other symptoms associated with the disease. In most cases, the benefits of the orchiectomy will be temporary, and eventually the disease will reassert itself. However, the procedure may stave off the effects of the disease for many months or years, during which the patient will experience a significantly improved quality of life. The operation is minor and can be performed on an outpatient basis in many cases.

There are shortcomings to this procedure. Many men find this surgery difficult to accept, even those who are no longer sexually active. To many, it strikes at the very heart of their manhood. These fears are understandable, but the imagination tends to exaggerate the consequences of the treatment. Although most men will experience some loss of libido following a bilateral orchiectomy, many men retain sexual function. Other than this, hot flashes are the only common side effect of the operation.

Another disadvantage of the bilateral orchiectomy is that it is irreversible. A small minority of men will have a form of prostate cancer that is hormonally independent, and will not respond to the procedure. These men will gain no benefit from the operation. However, it is possible to achieve the same effect with hormonal therapy using LHRH analogs. Many men prefer this non-surgical approach.

Estrogen Therapy

The administration of the female hormone, estrogen, to inhibit the production of testosterone was until recently the most common form of hormonal deprivation therapy. The orally taken drug known as diethylstilbestrol, or DES, is the most widely used form of estrogen. One tablet is taken three times a day. It is much cheaper than alternative medications.

Studies have shown DES to be at least as effective as orchiectomy for halting the progression of prostate cancer. However, there are a number of side effects of estrogen therapy. These include water retention, breast growth and tenderness (gynecomastia), nausea, and vomiting. Even more serious, estrogen therapy may result in severe circulatory problems, such as blood clots and stroke. DES administered in small doses (1 mg daily) seems to result in little loss of effectiveness and fewer cardiovascular complications. Nonetheless, estrogen therapy is seldom recommended for patients over 70 or in poor health.

LHRH Therapy

This recently developed therapy uses *leutinizing hormone releasing hormone* (LHRH) analogs, a synthesized form of a natural brain hormone. LHRH analogs effectively shut down production of testicular testosterone, achieving the same effect as bilateral orchiectomy, the surgical removal of the testicles. LHRH analogs can be taken by daily, self-administered injection or more preferably administered once a month by "depot" injection in the physician's office. The two LHRH analogs currently available in the U.S. are commercially named Lupron and Zoladex.

This new therapy has been a boon to those men who wish to avoid surgery or the unwanted side effects of estrogen therapy. However, it is not without its disadvantages. The drug is expensive ---- about $250 per month. This may be prohibitively high for some patients.

The side effects of LHRH analogs are the same as those of bilateral orchiectomy, namely hot flashes, some loss of libido, and in some cases impotence. Infrequent gastrointestinal side effects have been reported as well.

An unusual "flare reaction" is observed when LHRH therapy is initiated, causing a brief rise in testosterone level, and sub-sequent exacerbation of cancer symptoms, such as bone pain and urinary difficulties in some men. This initial phase lasts for only a week or two. Small doses of estrogen, or antiandrogens, such as flutimide, are sometimes administered previous to the initiation of LHRH therapy, and act to block this flare phenomenon.

Combination Therapy

This treatment combines the use of LHRH analogs (or orchiectomy) with an antiandrogen, used to block the small percentage of testosterone produced by the adrenal glands. Flutimide is the most commonly prescribed antiandrogen, and must be taken orally every 8 hours.

Recent studies have indicated that combination therapy is superior to other forms of hormonal therapy, extending the average period of remission by several months. Furthermore, the percentage of patients who respond to therapy is higher, and more experience complete remission of the disease. However, clinical evaluation has been contradictory concerning the advantages of combination therapy over monotherapy (the use of a single treatment to inhibit male hormone production). A 1990 National Cancer Institute study is currently under way to measure the advantages gained by combination therapy.

The side effects of flutimide vary. A significant number of men experience noticeable breast enlargement or tenderness, although typically to a lesser degree than with estrogen therapy. About 10% of patients experience diarrhea problems. Nausea and vomiting have also been reported. Flutimide has been known to affect liver function as well.

Chemotherapy

This is "chemical therapy," involving the use of potent chemical agents to kill cancer cells or interfere with their ability to grow and multiply. These drugs circulate throughout the body in the bloodstream, and often produce many unpleasant side effects. To minimize the harm these powerful drugs can do, dosages must be carefully regulated.

Chemotherapy is typically reserved for patients that do not respond or have become resistent to standard hormonal therapy. They may relieve symptoms of the disease in some men, but at this point, no anticancer agent has proven highly effective in the treatment of metastatic prostate cancer in a majority of cases.

Some of the different chemotherapy drugs currently used for the treatment of prostate cancer are listed below:

• CYTOTOXIC agents, of which several are available, are the standard treatment for forms of prostate cancer that do not respond to hormonal manipulation. Results have been disappointing, although this has been attributed to the very late stage at which most patients initiate cytotoxic chemotherapy. Attempts are being made to "target" cytotoxic agents to tumor sites, allowing for increased drug levels and cell death in cancer tissues while minimizing toxicity for healthy tissues.

• CYTADREN (aminoglutethimide), administered in combination with hydrocortisone, inhibits adrenal production of male hormones. Response rates in those that have failed initial hormonal therapy are generally poor, although a few patients have reacted very positively to this therapy.

• EMCYT (estramustine phostphate), which acts to combine the hormonal effects of estrogen with specific cell toxicity. No advantage over DES (estrogen) has been observed, although there is evidence of improved response in combination with other chemotherapy agents, such as Velban.

• NIZORAL (ketoconazole), an antifungal agent that inhibits male hormone production. Some positive results have been gained in those who have become resistent to standard hormonal therapy.

• PROGESTINS, such as hydroxyprogesterone caproate, megestrol acetate, and medrogestone, inhibit testosterone production, and have resulted in partial, temporary responses in some patients.

• SURAMIN, a growth factor inhibiting agent currently under investigation. The objective responses have not been impressive, although a few patients have responded well, and many experience a reduction in pain associated with bone cancer.

New chemical agents are continuously under development and testing. Several are unmentioned here because research findings into the efficacy of the agents have yet to be made public. With improved knowledge regarding the origins and development of prostate cancer, it is likely that new agents with improved therapeutic potential will soon be made available.

Chapter 8

EVALUATION OF TREATMENTS BY STAGE

We shall not cease from exploration
And the end of all our exploring
Will be to arrive where we started
And know the place for the first time."

T. S. Eliot

The most important factor to be considered for the management of prostate cancer is the stage. However, it is not the only relevant factor to be considered in selecting an appropriate form of therapy. Assessment of the malignant potential of a tumor, based on tumor volume, grade of disease, DNA ploidy analysis, and change over time in prostate specific antigen (PSA) levels in the blood are all pertinent factors a physician must consider in forming his prognosis. For a patient whose cancer the doctor deems unlikely to become a health problem during his lifetime, careful observation and follow-up will often be preferable to any immediate treatment.

The age and health of the patient must also be taken into account. Prostate cancer is usually a slowly developing cancer, and men may live a decade or more with no detrimental impact from the disease. For some men, the benefit from therapy is minimal, and may be far outweighed by the potentially harmful ramifications of therapy.

The concern of the patient to avoid severe complications may become an important criterion in the selection of a treatment as well. Ideally, the physician will form a treatment plan to minimize the impact of the disease while sparing the patient undesirable side effects of therapy.

Treatment of prostate cancer by radical prostatectomy, external radiation therapy, and various forms of hormonal therapy has been ongoing for decades. A mass of statistical data has been collected to analyze the effect of these therapies with the intent of improving treatment. Unfortunately, most studies done to date are non-randomized and suffer from a variety of uncontrolled conditions that significantly complicate evaluation of the information. Testing methods used to determine the effectiveness of treatment vary, as do staging methods prior to therapy. Many factors may be used to assess outcome: 5, 10 and 15-year survival rates, disease-free survival, time to

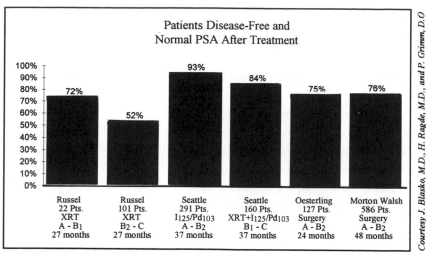

Figure 11. Comparison of prostate cancer treatments using the PSA test as an indicator or treatment effectiveness. Number of patients, form of treatment, and the stages treated are shown. Average follow-up period is shown in months.

progression, and time to recurrence have all been used in reports analyzing the effect of therapy. Improvements in staging techniques and treatments also contribute to the difficulty of measuring the role and value of different therapies. Few multidisciplinary randomized clinical trials have been completed to clarify these data.

The use of the PSA test to indicate the return or progression of disease offers a new means of comparing the available forms of therapy, especially in the short term. This gives physicians a means of evaluating not only conventional treatments, but also more recently developed alternative treatments. But because prostate cancer is slow growing in most instances, long-term follow-up is necessary to fully assess the value of any therapy. At this point, little information is available for most of these newer forms of treatment.

STAGE A1: focalized lower grade impalpable tumors

The vast majority ---- about 85 to 90% ---- of stage A1 prostate cancers will not become health or life threatening during the lifetime of the patient. Usually discovered following a transurethral resection of the prostate (TURP), these small tumors seldom demand any treatment other than careful monitoring. Only men under 60 might be considered at appreciable risk of disease progression. Those whose cancer shows aneuploid characteristics upon DNA ploidy analysis may also be at greater risk (*see Evaluation and Staging, p. 64*).

Among treatments for A1 patients, a repeat TURP is occasionally used. The value of this procedure is questionable. Although hormonal therapy is typically reserved for late stage patients, one study shows that combination therapy may be an effective curative treatment for stage A patients. It should be considered by those men who are uncomfortable with the idea of doing nothing to treat their cancer.

Studies have shown no apparent value in aggressive treatment of stage A1 prostate cancer. In fact, an examination of radical prostatectomy specimens at the University of Utah in 51% of cases found no remaining presence of disease! Radical surgery is now typically considered inappropriate therapy for stage A1 patients.

Stage A2: high-grade or diffuse impalpable tumors

Clinically diagnosed stage A2 carcinoma of the prostate is a more aggressive form of cancer than stage A1 carcinoma, and possesses a propensity to metastisize. For this reason, it will usually merit some form of immediate treatment.

In as many as 25% of cases, disease will already be found to have spread to the lymph nodes when a lymphadenectomy is performed. The likelihood of spread to the lymph nodes is closely related to the grade of tumor. In one study, 0% of those with a Gleason score of 2-4 possessed positive lymph nodes, whereas 75% of those with a Gleason score of 8-10 had lymph node involvement. Although little data is available on untreated A2 disease, those with low-grade A2 tumors are possible candidates for deferred treatment and close observation.

Treatments of stage A2 prostate cancer include radical prostatectomy, external-beam radiation therapy, and brachytherapy. Analysis of radical prostatectomy specimens has shown that something between 30% and 50% of patients will have extension of the cancer beyond the confines of the prostate, and thus cannot be said to be cured by the operation. However, this does not mean that the cancer will necessarily recur (*see Treatment Failure and Recurrence, p. 111*). Ironically, those most amenable to cure with surgery — low grade, low volume tumors, likely to be confined to the prostate — are also those who will least benefit from the operation. Additional hormonal or radiation therapy is often used in instances where evidence suggests that the cancer has not been completely excised. Even taking into account the fairly high level of incomplete excision of the cancer, results with prostatectomy have been good, with about two-thirds of patients alive and free of disease at 10 years, and only 10% dying from cancer. This appears superior to the 'watch and wait' approach of expectant management.

Radiation therapy has achieved results roughly equivelent to radical prostatectomy. However, there is some evidence that those undergoing radiation therapy are at a slightly greater risk of local recurrence than those who undergo surgical treatment. Evidence exists that many if not most men treated with radiation therapy will have residual cancer, but disease progression may not occur for a decade or more. Thus, for younger men, aged 40 to 65, radical prostatectomy yeilds a somewhat better prognosis in the long run. On the other hand, some believe that those unlikely to have cancer confined to the prostate may be better treated with radiation therapy than with prostatectomy.

Radioactive seed implantation has also demonstrated an ability to control cancer in stage A2 patients roughly equal to results obtained with external-beam radiation therapy. Iodine-125 has been the most common radioactive source used for patients with this stage of disease, and has resulted in a very low percentage of complications due to treatment. Iodine-125's slow rate of decay makes its use most appropriate for cancers with a Gleason score under 7. In cases of high grade cancer, Palladium-103 should in theory be a more effective radiation source. Improvements in implantation techniques allow for more accurate placement of seeds using ultrasound guidance than the older manual implantation method. Five-year data using the new technique is very promising (*see p. 104*), even though longer-term data on the effectiveness of this form of brachytherapy is not yet available.

Stage B1: Focalized palpable tumor confined to one lobe

Stage B1 cancer seems in many ways less aggressive than A2 carcinoma of the prostate. Moderate or high grade B1 cancer is less likely to have extended to the lymph nodes than in A2 cancer. This is an encouraging finding, since those who are discovered to have lymph node or seminal vesicle involvement have a significantly worse prognosis.

Aggressive treatment may be most advantageous to patients presenting with B1 tumor, since the chances of cure are good, and in most cases the disease will eventually become life-threatening without treatment. However, men in their eighties are candidates for careful observation and deferred treatment. The life expectancy for an 80-year-old male is about 7 years, and findings indicate that only about one-third of B1 cancers will progress at 6 years after diagnosis. Those who do progress will often live several more years. Thus, rarely will an 80-year-old die of his stage B1 prostate cancer. Men in their seventies with small low grade B1 tumors are also good candidates for observation, especially if health mitigates against aggressive treatment.

The effectiveness of radical prostatectomy in treating B1 prostate cancer is well established. Two-thirds or more of those receiving the operation will live 10 years without recurrence. Only 15-20% will die from recurrence within 15 years. Men with stage B1 prostate cancer are ideal candidates for the Walsh nerve-sparing technique, which has been able to preserve potency in about 67% of men under the age of 70.

Radiation therapy and brachytherapy have shown similar therapeutic effects, although definitive cure is less easily demonstrated with these treatments. Nonetheless, each form of therapy shows survival rates approaching the survival rate in men of an equivelent age without prostate cancer.

Stage B2: Palpable tumor involving over half of prostate

Stage B2 carcinoma of the prostate is the most advanced stage of cancer still clinically confined to the prostate gland. Treatment of stage B2 prostate cancer is complicated by the difficulty in clinically assessing whether the cancer has penetrated the prostatic capsule, in which case it should be classified as stage C prostate cancer. There is a very large incidence of understaging in clinically diagnosed B2 cancer, as evidenced by examination of prostatectomy specimens. Studies indicate as high as 60% of patients diagnosed with B2 prostate cancer will actually have stage C (cancer extending beyond prostate capsule) or stage D1 (positive lymph nodes) cancer upon microscopic examination of surgical specimens. Tumor size may be the best predictor of those who have cancer no longer confined to the prostate. Extension of cancer beyond the prostate is found in the vast majority of those with tumors exceeding 10 cubic centimeters, compared with only about 10% of those with tumors under 4 cc. Most disturbing are data suggesting that as many as half of B2 patients will have microscopic invasion of the seminal vesicles by cancer, which correlates closely with recurrence of the cancer after treatment.

As one might expect from this information, stage B2 patients undergoing radical prostatectomy have not fared as well as stage B1 patients. The nerve sparing technique fared poorly in one sample group, with only one-quarter of patients having both complete removal of tumor and preservation of potency. More than a fourth of patients failed both complete excision of the tumor and preservation of potency, thus bringing into question the value of the procedure for the majority of patients. Even so, one study shows about half will survive 10 years with no recurrence of the cancer. Even among those that eventually suffer recurrence, many will live beyond this 10-year threshold.

Radiation therapy has generated similar 5 and 10 year results. However, local failure seems to be somewhat higher, and recurrence of cancer may continue to occur beyond 10 years, indicating that cure may be less likely. Radioactive seed implantation with I-125 has failed to maintain local control of the disease in patients with stage B2 prostate cancer, resulting in a higher incidence of recurrence at 5 and 10 years after treatment. High grade cancer responded particularly poorly to this form of therapy. More recent results using the newly developed implantation techniques and palladium seeds have proven more successful. A five-year study by the Northwest Tumor Institute in Seattle has followed 472 patients with radioactive seed implantation, the great majority with stage B carcinoma. Eighty-seven percent of patients are free of disease and have PSA levels within the normal range. A similar study of 230 patients treated with surgery reported an 82% disease-free survival rate at 5 years. Using PSA testing as a measure of treatment effectiveness, ultrasound-guided brachytherapy has compared very favorably with other forms of treatment (*see Fig. 11 on p. 97*).

Combining radiation therapy with hormonal therapy prior to and during irradiation has achieved a lower incidence of local failure in patients with stage B2 cancer than with external radiation therapy alone. However, many physicians have expressed concern that hormonal treatment may reduce the radiosensitivity of cancer cells. As a consequence, it has been suggested that hormonal therapy should be halted 30-60 days prior to radiation therapy or implantation of radioisotopes. Several studies are under way to test the effect of combination hormonal therapy with other forms of therapy.

Stage C: Tumor no longer confined to prostate

The treatment of this stage presents many difficulties, since prostate cancer is presumed by most physicians to be incurable once it has extended beyond the prostate gland. Thus many use hormonal therapy to treat the symptoms of the disease, and to slow its progression. Since the tumor may have penetrated the prostatic capsule, but does not appear to have metastisized, curative methods have been used to treat patients with stage C disease as well.

Radical prostatectomy has proven ineffective in treating stage C patients. Half or more of those with stage C have tumorous pelvic lymph nodes upon dissection and examination, and will not benefit from the operation. Of those that undergo the operation, about 20% will have been over-staged and actually possess stage B2 disease, which may be cured by procedure. Most will not be cured by radical prostatectomy alone, but may benefit from the removal of the main tumor. The treatment does appear to improve survival.

Combining other therapies with radical prostatectomy seem to improve the results obtained with surgery. External beam irradiation immediately following surgery or at recurrence of cancer has acheived positive results in several studies. Radioactive implantation for those who are at high risk for recurrence after surgery has also been used with some success. These methods await further investigation.

Attempts have been made to "downstage" those diagnosed with stage C cancer using 3-6 months of combination hormonal therapy prior to surgery. This therapy usually significantly shrinks the tumor, and the majority upon digital examination appear to have downstaged to B stage tumor. However, examination of surgical specimens from most of these patients still show extension of prostate cancer beyond the capsule or at the point of surgical resection. The overall impact of attempts to downstage the disease remain unclear, and should be further explored.

External beam radiation therapy is the most effective lone therapy in treatment of stage C, especially in cases where invasion of the seminal vesicles is suspected. Radiation therapy using mixed photon-neutron beam has shown superior results to standard x-ray irradiation. Combining low dose radioactive seed implantation with radiation therapy has achieved similar beneficial results to radiation therapy. Radioactive seed implantation used as the sole therapy has resulted in high recurrence rates, and does not appear to be an ideal treatment in stage C patients.

Combination hormonal therapy in those that are poor candidates for more aggressive treatment has shown very good local control of the disease in stage C patients. Tumor shrinkage is considerable, and time to progression is extended over those who receive no treatment at all. Combination hormonal therapy has been more effective than any form of hormonal monotherapy in achieving these results. In addition, the likelihood of alleviating urinary symptoms of the disease with hormonal therapy is very good.

Stage D1: Metastatic disease that has extended to the pelvic lymph nodes

Of those with stage D1 prostate cancer, most will develop bone metastases within five years without treatment. Likelihood of cure is very small, hence most treatments prescribed for stage D1 patients are used to reduce symptoms or to extend time to disease progression. Those with minimal pelvic lymph node involvement have a better prognosis than those who have extensive lymph node metastases.

Radical prostatectomy with extended lymph node dissection in an attempt to remove the bulk of the disease has resulted in mild success in some patients. This has shown best results in those patients with low volume prostate tumors and minimal pelvic lymph node involvement. In others, the treatment is unlikely to be of much benefit.

Combining radical surgery with hormonal manipulation has had improved results over surgery alone. A study indicates that patients with stage D1 prostate cancer who receive immediate orchiectomies following surgical removal of the prostate have improved survival in carefully selected patients. The Mayo series reported an 87% survival at 10 years. However, many patients will not be good candidates for this treatment.

Radiation therapy is effective in only a small percentage of cases. Radiation therapy has been largely unsuccessful when used as an adjuvant therapy after radical surgery. Fifty percent of patients undergoing such treatment will have bone metastases in five years, which is not a great improvement over observation alone.

Because radioactive seed implantation is limited to the prostate itself, brachytherapy has had generally poor results with stage D1 patients.

Hormonal therapy has had good results in reducing symptoms and extending the time to progression, when bone metastases appear. Debate in the medical community currently focuses on whether hormonal therapy should be undertaken prior to the appearance of bone metastases or should be delayed. Whether a survival advantage is imparted with early hormonal therapy is unclear at this point. Younger patients and those with high grade tumor do seem to benefit from early initiation of hormonal therapy.

Patients receiving combination hormonal therapy using LHRH agonists and the anti-androgen flutimide show a greater level of response than those who receive monotherapy that achieves only partial androgen blockage. Orchiectomy combined with an anti-androgen would be likely to obtain a similar result.

Stage D2: Distant metastatic disease

In those who have stage D2 prostate cancer, the disease has spread to the bones, or in some cases, soft tissue organs other than the prostate. Rarely is cure attainable in patients with advanced prostate cancer, and in large part treatment focuses on alleviation of the symptoms ---- typically, aches and pain in the bones of the back and hips.

Hormonal therapy is the conventional form of treatment for men with stage D2 prostate cancer. There is no question about the beneficial impact this form of treatment has on the vast majority of men with advanced prostate cancer. Pain and other symptoms are often dramatically reduced, and an objective response in reduction of tumor burden is usually seen as well.

Many different forms of hormonal therapy are in use. Orchiectomy, LHRH analogs, estrogens, and others have all achieved striking results.

Combination hormonal therapy arguably provides the greatest benefit to the patient. This is because no single hormone-blocking agent can completely shut off production of tostesterone, which the cancer requires to grow. But combination hormonal therapy, which combines a LHRH analog, such as leuprolide, with an anti-androgen, such as flutimide, can achieve total blockage of testosterone. Although study results have been somewhat contradictory, it appears that combination therapy provides a small but significant life-prolonging benefit over forms of monotherapy. For those who poorly tolerate the drug flutimide or cannot afford the high cost of combination hormonal therapy, megestrol plus low-dose estrogen may provide an alternate means of attaining total androgen blockade.

In the great majority of cases, the cancer will initially respond to hormonal therapy, and may be kept in remission for several years, but eventually the patient will relapse. At that point, some response to another form of hormonal treatment may be achieved for a briefer period of time. Eventually a patient will cease to respond to hormonal therapy. Many doctors take their patients off hormonal therapy once progression of the disease occurs, but there is evidence that hormonal therapy even after relapse may maintain partial control over the cancer. Several forms of chemotherapy are currently under clinical evaluation for use on those who have relapsed under hormonal therapy.

Radiation therapy is sometimes used in late stage patients to relieve pain, however, the side effects of radiation therapy can be as bad as the condition it is used to treat. As a palliative therapy, external-beam radiation should be resorted to only after hormonal therapy has failed. Partical beam radiation therapy is presently under investigation, and may be able to directly target metastatic tumors without the significant side effects of conventional radiation therapy. Strontium^{89} chloride is a radiopharmaceutical recently approved for marketing by the FDA. Once injected, it goes directly to the sites of metastatic bone disease to relieve pain symptoms. It is effective for several months in most cases, with few side-effects when compared with narcotic substances or external radiation.

Treatment Failure and Recurrence

Treatment failure means a form of therapy has proven unsuccessful in eliminating the cancer or maintaining control over the growth of the disease. In evaluating treatment failure, physicians examine whether the failure was "local" — the return of cancer in the area of the prostate — or "distant" — the appearance or growth of metastases at sites distant from the prostate, where the disease originated.

For a curative treatment for prostate cancer, local failure and recurrence are more likely when there is evidence that the cancer has not been completely eradicated in the vicinity of the prostate. In the case of a radical prostatectomy, examination of the surgical specimen may show that the cancer extends beyond the capsule of the prostate, the seminal vesicles are infected, or the presence of cancer at the point of resection where the surgeon cut across the urethra and surrounding tissue to remove the prostate. About 40-45% of radical prostatectomy patients exhibit one or more of these conditions, all strong indicators that some cancer remains in the patient. In such cases, a patient is at higher risk of local failure and recurrence of his disease. A positive biopsy 12 or more months after treatment is a strong indicator of increased risk for local failure after either radiation therapy or brachytherapy. An elevated PSA level following therapy is perhaps the best predictor of the eventual return of the disease.

Evidence that the cancer has not been eliminated after curative therapy does not always mean the disease will recur. In a significant number of cases, there may be no observed regrowth of the original tumor or appearance of distant metastases. Studies suggest that less than 30% of stage B patients who have evidence of incomplete removal of cancer following a radical prostatectomy will suffer relapse during a follow-up period of 5 years or more. Similarly, one study showed that about 20% of patients with positive biopsies following radiation therapy showed no recurrence of the disease for 10 years or more.

When local failure does occur, the likelihood of distant failure, or the development of metastatic disease, is greatly increased. About two-thirds of those that show local failure subsequently develop metastatic disease. Additional therapy can be used immediately following initial treatment for those that appear to be at risk of recurrence, or may be withheld until after the disease has reappeared. There are two goals of additional therapy: reduction of the likelihood of distant failure, and alleviation of symptoms that become manifest with the return of the disease.

The common forms of additional therapy prescribed for those at risk for local failure after surgery are radiation therapy or hormonal therapy. Radiation therapy immediately following surgery has been shown to significantly reduce the chance of local recurrence, but it is unclear if it reduces the likelihood that patients will develop metastatic disease. There are some complications of this additional therapy, but these may be limited by allowing the patient to heal from surgery before beginning radiation treatments. Hormonal treatment has had very good results in preventing recurrence in patients at increased risk of treatment failure with few complications.

Additional therapy may be used once the cancer has returned. "Salvage" prostatectomies performed on patients following failed radiation therapy have resulted in a high level of severe complications with no clear advantage to the patient, and are therefore not recommended. Radiation therapy applied once cancer has recurred in prostatectomy patients can have temporary benefits, but is not as successful as radiation therapy used immediately after prostatectomy. There is little information on the effectiveness of a salvage prostatectomy following brachytherapy, although presumably there would be a greater risk of complications due to radiation-caused tissue damage and scarring in the area of the prostate.

Hormonal therapy after recurrence has been very effective in halting the progression of disease for many years. Most of the patients who receive hormonal treatment after treatment failure will eventually relapse. At that point, a secondary form of hormonal therapy is often prescribed, and many patients will initially respond for a period before relapsing again. Once a patient has ceased to respond to hormonal treatment of any kind, one of several kinds of chemotherapy may be used. Chemotherapy has not proven particularly effective in a majority of patients with prostate cancer. It is hoped that in the near future, more effective chemotherapeutic agents will be developed to treat patients who no longer respond to hormonal therapy.

Lies, Damn Lies and Statistics

The information provided in this chapter seeks to summarize and evaluate state-of-the-art treatment for prostate cancer in the U.S. To make this evaluation by stage, findings of the past 20 years have been weighed for relevance and accuracy. A great effort has been made to give a balanced presentation, based on current knowledge.

But this is not the final word.

Although the statistics above provide a general picture of what the patient may expect from treatment, they may not be representative of present success rates. Over the past handful of years, steady improvements in all fields have increased the effectiveness of treatment. Furthermore, several techniques now under investigation are not included in this analysis, but may offer definite advantages to some men. It is possible that some of these new therapies may in years to come supplant the conventional treatments of today.

Finally, statistics are general. But as an individual, you are unique. And your case is just as unique. This is especially true when dealing with a disease as unpredictable as prostate cancer. What is true of most men may not be true for you.

Even in a worst case scenario, there is reason for hope. Lloyd Ney, founder of PAACT, a patient advocacy organization for prostate cancer, was diagnosed with late stage D2 prostate cancer, and given only six months to live. He traveled to Canada to undergo combination hormonal therapy ---- then unavailable in the U.S. He went into total remission, and within months, the cancer was undetectable! Over eight years later, he is still going strong, and working to help others who find themselves in a similar predicament.

Although his physician had written him off, he didn't give up hope. Neither should you.

Chapter 9

✖ FITNESS, DIET, AND NUTRITION

"Natural forces within us are the true healers of disease."

Hippocrates

Good health is a universal concern. But it becomes a critical concern for anyone whose physical well-being has been threatened by a serious disease. For those men who have always striven to take care of themselves, prostate cancer can drive them to the fatalistic attitude that a healthy lifestyle is without value. Others, who have paid only superficial attention to their health, may require a health crisis before they develop true appreciation for the blessings of good health. In either case, it is all too easy for a man with prostate cancer to slip into a dejected unconcern for his physical care, and rather than looking out for his health, spend his time looking back in misery on "the good old days" when his body was sound and well.

Fortunately, it is never too late to adopt health-promoting strategies. Every man with prostate cancer, whether undergoing medical treatment or electing to take a stance of "watchful waiting," can take decisive action to improve his condition. Men who take steps to improve their health not only significantly enhance the likelihood of successful treatment, but are also better able to tolerate the side-effects of therapy. For men who make the effort, the reward is an improved quality of life. And men who take an active role in combating their prostate cancer will gain the emotional satisfaction of knowing they are participating in their own healing process.

If you have prostate cancer — or wish to take positive steps to avoid the disease — keep this in mind: the body is an amazing machine, of such incredible complexity that modern science has achieved only rudimentary knowledge of its processes. Unlike any man-made machine, the body is constantly, aggressively acting to repair itself and eliminate anything that is a threat to its normal, healthy processes. A physician may aid the body's healing in any number of ways, but only the body itself has the power to restore and sustain health. Yet like any other machine, the body requires suitable care and maintenance to continue proper functioning. Like a finely tuned racing car, the body needs the proper fuel to run well: this means a balanced diet and a good supply of essential nutrients. Rest and exercise are important parts of the body's maintenance program. As the caretaker of your own body, you are in control of the quality of care your body receives.

Overcoming prostate cancer places great demands on the body. Yet you have the power to shore up your body's defenses against the disease! The major sections of this appendix aim to provide general guidelines and current information on the self-help methods you can undertake to promote your body's health and healing.

Getting Fit For The Fight addresses general physical fitness and its benefits.

Diet and Prostate Cancer examines the scientific evidence that links diet and prostate cancer, and gives general recommendations for the prevention or treatment of cancer of the prostate.

Nutritional Supplements surveys the recent findings associating the use of vitamin and mineral supplements with cancer treatment and prevention.

Getting Fit For The Fight

The fitness craze of the eighties awakened the country to the importance of exercise as part of a healthy lifestyle. But the eighties are over and as we've grown older, age has conferred upon us a host of aches, pains, stiff joints and sore backs that interfere with our capacity to remain as athletically active as we once were. Busy schedules, boredom with exercise, and medical ailments — among them prostate cancer — can also get in the way of physical activity. As a consequence, many of us have slipped back into sedentary ways — those of us who ever left them to begin with!

But if the years have convinced you that fitness is better left to the young, think again! The benefits of exercise are greater now than at any time in your life. If you've left exercise behind, take advantage of those benefits by becoming physically active again. A fit body is a great ally in the battle against prostate cancer.

Some of the physical benefits of a daily routine of exercise include:

- An improved cardiovascular system, a more efficient digestive system, and a more active metabolism.

- Reduced body fat, a lower level of cholesterol, and improved muscle tone.

- A fit body with greater regenerative powers, more able to cope with the side-effects of the cancer and therapy.

- Reduced perception of pain and physical ailments.

- More energy and a better appetite.

- Improved sleep patterns.

- A strengthened immune system.

- A greater sense of physical well-being.

Beyond the physical advantages of becoming fit, there are also compelling mental and emotional benefits of regular exercise. Exercise is a great way to relieve tension and reduce stress. Regular exercise is also an effective means to combat the negative emotions that assault the prostate cancer patient. Endorphins released by strenuous activity act to naturally relieve frustration, calm anxieties, stimulate mental alertness, and lift the spirits. Prostate cancer and its treatment can effect your body image and sense of self-esteem. Getting fit will help restore lost confidence, and return to you a level of mastery over your own body.

Developing a Fitness Program

No matter what your age or physical condition, there is a fitness program right for you. Yet some of you may be hesitant to read on. Perhaps you've already devised some ready excuse for why you should not commit yourself to a regular fitness program.

This is understandable. Many men, especially those that have not made exercise a regular feature of their daily lives, associate physical fitness with unpleasant images and experiences: burning lungs, aching joints, and cramping muscles, not to mention just plain weariness and drudgery. Some men fear that they will injure themselves, or wish to avoid aggravating their prostate. Some simply believe their poor condition makes it impossible to engage in any kind of strenuous physical activity.

Fortunately, you aren't required to become the next Charles Atlas! Virtually everyone is able to take up light-to-moderate exercise of some kind — without the need to worry that becoming fit means hours of boredom, pain and fatigue. In fact, most active people derive real enjoyment from exercise. The worst part is beginning. Once you've established a regular fitness regimen, you'll find that over time the unpleasant aspects of exercise diminish while the enjoyable qualities increase. That means you're getting in shape!

Here are some important rules you should observe when you adopt a new exercise program:

Rule 1: Always consult your doctor. Once you have a fitness program you'd like to try — or if you want advice in forming a program that fits your interests, condition and physical limitations — speak to your physician. He is in the best position to know what activities might pose a health risk to you. If your doctor gives the okay, go to it. Should you desire further guidance, ask your physician if he can refer you to a qualified physical therapist who will understand your special needs.

After you've begun a regular fitness program, you will probably experience a minor degree of muscle soreness and some fatigue, especially if it has been a long time since you engaged in strenuous activity. This is normal and should decline as your general level of conditioning improves. However, if you experience any acute pain, or if a chronic ache develops in some part of the body, you should temporarily halt exercising until you can consult with your physician concerning the problem.

Rule 2: Start slowly and gradually build up. If you try to do too much too fast, you run the risk of placing excessive demands on your body. This is true even for those who are already fit and active. Overconfidence when trying an exercise routine with which your body is unfamiliar can result in injury. At the very least, you may end up extremely sore and somewhat dispirited. You might lose a few days while your body recovers, and you may even prematurely abandon your fitness program. If you're not in shape, start out *very* lightly. It is advisable to always maintain a level of physical exertion well within your limits.

Over time, gradually increase your level of activity. Don't push yourself. It may take several weeks to show significant improvement. If your body seems to be handling your current degree of activity, do a little more and see how your body responds. Progress takes time, so keep your fitness regimen within your comfort zone.

Rule 3: Be consistent. If you don't exercise on a regular basis, you are unlikely to reap the rewards of physical fitness. You'll want to exercise several times a week to get results. Consistency is more important than the vigor of your exercise routine, so make every effort to keep on schedule. Any progress you make in conditioning your body can easily erode if you don't stick with it.

Don't try to make up for missed days. Getting in shape is an incremental process; you won't make any quick jumps in condition by exercising hard for just one day. You will only end up overdoing it. In fact, if you have missed a week or two, you probably need to reduce your routine a bit until you get back into the swing of things.

Even if you don't see any immediate progress, stay committed to your exercise program. Over time, your body will adapt as it becomes accustomed to your changed level of activity. If you stay with it for at least six weeks, you should notice very distinct improvements in the way your body functions. And in all likelihood, you'll discover that on a day-to-day basis, you feel better, too!

Rule 4: Get plenty of rest. Once you've raised your level of physical activity, you may find you need additional rest to restore your energy. To avoid depleting your body of resources that are desperately needed for your battle against cancer, make sure you get plenty of sleep on a regular basis.

However, just as you should avoid too much exercise, watch out that you don't get too much rest! Many men with prostate cancer struggle with chronic fatigue. The disease and several of its treatments can produce a feeling of lingering exhaustion. Stress and depression resulting from the disease are also debilitating. But oversleeping in response may only worsen the fatigue. Too much bed rest often leads to a state of lethargy, as your metabolism slows down and you become less and less active.

Combined, rest and exercise are effective weapons against fatigue. This is because rest and exercise work synergistically: the physical benefits of each can only be maximized in conjunction with the other. When a consistent daily balance is struck between rest and exercise, their effect is not exhaustion but a remarkable energizing of body and mind. Finding the proper balance of rest and exercise will make you fitter, healthier and happier. So don't neglect either one.

Rule 5: Find ways to make your exercise enjoyable. Exercise doesn't have to be dull and repetitive. If you can, find forms of exercise that you really enjoy. Recreational activities such as tennis, golf, swimming and biking can be a valuable part of a fitness regimen. Do your exercising in environments that you find stimulating. You might like the convenience of the local spa, where you can exercise and then take a pleasant dip in the pool or relax in the Jacuzzi. If you enjoy nature, go on hikes. Be creative. If you like fishing, take a brisk walk along the shoreline of a favorite fishing spot, stopping periodically for a few casts. You'll get some exercise and might come home with dinner as well!

Recommendations for an Effective Exercise Program

• Begin your exercise routine with a warm-up, involving stretching exercises and light calisthenics. Stretching before and after exercise is an important factor in maintaining flexibility and avoiding injury.

• Exercise at least three days a week. Daily exercise is preferable if possible. A daily fitness plan will help you to establish a consistent routine, and will better habituate your body to your higher level of activity.

• Exercise sessions should be at least 20 to 30 minutes of sustained activity to have a significant impact on your physical condition. This may be too stressful when you first start out. If necessary, begin at 5 or 10 minutes and build up your strength and endurance.

• To improve your cardiovascular condition, you need to raise your heart rate during exercise. This can be accomplished with a variety of aerobic exercises, such as brisk walking, jogging, bicycling, swimming, and, naturally, aerobics. Water aerobics are designed to reduce the body stress of aerobic exercises, and are ideal for older subjects. You should try to raise your heart rate to a level appropriate to your age and condition. If your heart begins to race, slow down. Men with heart conditions need to be especially cautious about this.

• If you work out at a gym, focus on doing exercises with light weight and high repetitions. This will tone your muscles and also provide some aerobic activity.

• Maintain a healthy nutritious diet with plenty of calories. You'll have a hard time getting your body to perform without sufficient fuel.

• Balance exercise with R & R. A relaxing pastime can be especially pleasurable right after strenuous activity. Reward yourself for your efforts to get in shape. Also make sure to get plenty of sleep so your body can fully recuperate, and be primed and ready for more.

• Include in your routine exercises that target on the prostate. These include squats, pelvic thrusts, and Kegel exercises, which are typically used to treat incontinence problems (see p. 169). These exercises will improve the muscle tone of the tissues surrounding the prostate gland and increase blood flow to the region.

• When you begin to lose interest, remind yourself of the many rewards of exercise: an improved appearance, more energy, better general health, and a more positive state of mind. If they could put the benefits of exercise in a pill, it would surely be the world's best known miracle drug! So never forget that by keeping yourself fit you are assisting your body in its fight against prostate cancer.

Diet and Prostate Cancer

A healthy diet is central to a healthy lifestyle. We know this is true because we hear it every day. We are bombarded with this message on TV, in the newspapers, in conversation, and on the labels of the products we buy. All stress the importance of good nutrition. Yet how many of us actually eat the way we should?

Despite these daily reminders, the diet of the average American male is high in fat, low in fiber, and overly reliant on "junk food," which contains little or no nutritional value. In contrast, the current USDA recommendations suggest a diet high in fiber, low in fat, and rich in complex carbohydrates, with plenty of whole grains, fruits, and vegetables. Failure to maintain healthy eating habits is now recognized as a major factor in the health problems of our nation.

Based on studies of incidence, a close connection between cancer and diet has long been suspected. And now there is a growing body of evidence confirming this close link between diet and cancer — including prostate cancer. In fact, existing scientific data indicates that other than an individual's genetic make-up, no factor has greater influence on a man's likelihood of developing prostate cancer in later life than his diet.

Fortunately, recent research also demonstrates that dietary habits can improve the prognosis of a man already diagnosed with prostate cancer, regardless of stage. So it's never too late to change unhealthy ways. Given what we know now, it makes sense for every man with prostate cancer to increase his chances for recovery by adopting a healthier diet.

General Dietary Guidelines

There is no definitive diet for preventing or treating prostate cancer. What specific changes to diet should be recommended may depend on the individual concerned. It is always best to consult one's physician or a qualified nutritionist for help in developing an individualized diet. It is important to note that there is no evidence that diet alone can cure prostate cancer, so no one should attempt to use it as a substitute for medical treatment. However, in general, there are steps a man with prostate cancer can and should take to enhance his prospects for overcoming this disorder.

Eat A Low-Fat Diet

The average American man gets about 36% of his total calories from fat in his diet. Yet the American Cancer Society recommends reducing total fat intake to no more than 30% of total calories for all men and women, including cancer patients. Numerous studies have implicated excessive fat consumption with the development of cancer. Limiting dietary fat may be especially

important in retarding the development of prostate cancer. Statistical studies have established a
link between prostate cancer and a high-fat diet.
Incidence of prostate cancer is highest in coun-
tries where high-fat diets are prevalent. Prostate
cancer is considerably less common among Asian
men than men in the U.S., yet Asian-Americans
who have adopted a typical American diet have
an incidence of prostate cancer closely approaching
other Americans.

Studies also show a connection between fat in
the diet and mortality rates from prostate cancer.
A study from the Harvard School of Public Health
in 1993 found that men with prostate cancer who
ate high-fat diets had a 79% greater chance of developing advanced cases. This risk doubled when
the fat came from red meat.

Thus, the most effective way to reduce your
risk is to cut down on animal fat in your diet. Always get lean meat and don't eat red meat more
than once per week at most. Instead, eat white fish
and skinless poultry. Limit your consumption of
dairy products. Also avoid saturated fats and
heavy oils, such as butter, margarine, shortening
and corn oil. Instead, favor polyunsaturated oils in
cooking, such as olive, peanut, canola, linseed
and safflower oils. Keep an eye out for heavily
processed foods, fast foods and snack foods, all of
which are usually high in fat.

It is also notable that the percentage of body
fat, not just fats consumed in foods, may contribute to the growth of prostate cancer. According to

the American Cancer Society, overweight people have roughly twice the cancer mortality rate of people who aren't overweight. Obesity also complicates surgery for prostate cancer, may contribute to symptoms of the disease, and increases the likelihood of heart disease and other health problems. All in all, men who are significantly overweight would do well to reduce their level of body fat.

Reduce Cholesterol To Healthy Levels

In the popular mind, cholesterol has come to be seen as a deadly substance, but in reality most cholesterol is manufactured by the body itself for the building of cellular membranes and the formation of vital hormones. The dangers associated with cholesterol occur when supply exceeds demand. Excess cholesterol has been strongly linked to heart attacks and strokes, and may contribute to impotence problems in some men. And although experimental evidence is inconclusive, there is some reason to suspect high cholesterol also plays a role in prostate cancer.

A cholesterol level that exceeds 240 milligrams per deciliter (mg/dl) signals danger. But the component elements of one's blood cholesterol are also relevant. Cholesterol comes in two forms: low-density lipoproteins (LDLs) and high-density lipoproteins. Research shows that low levels of high density lipoproteins (HDL's) may pose as great a health risk as high total cholesterol levels. It now appears that higher than average levels of

HDL cholesterol can reduce the odds of future health problems. In general, it is wise for men with prostate cancer to reduce their cholesterol levels to around 180 to 200 mg/dl, while maintaining HDL levels at about 45 mg/dl or higher.

Intuitively, it would seem the best way to reduce your cholesterol level would be to eat foods low in cholesterol. But dietary cholesterol has surprisingly little impact on blood cholesterol. There is however a close relationship between dietary fat and the level of serum (blood) cholesterol. Once again, saturated fats are the major offender. Reducing fat intake is the most effective means to lower cholesterol through diet. Substitution of monounsaturated fats for saturated fats will help to lower LDL levels while maintaining the level of HDL's in your bloodstream.

Accompanying dietary changes can also have an impact on cholesterol levels. Most evidence shows that added fiber in the diet can noticeably lower cholesterol. It is generally a good idea to reduce one's dietary cholesterol from meat and dairy sources to 300 mg/day or less. This is about as much cholesterol as you will find in twelve ounces of ground beef, six ounces of steamed shrimp, or one and a half eggs. Surprisingly, moderate levels of alcohol consumption — a couple of drinks a day — seems to raise HDL levels, which may account for the lower rates of heart disease among those who drink wine with their dinner compared with those who abstain from drinking.

Another important factor is exercise, which can boost HDL levels by as much as 10% to 20%. In contrast, smoking can reduce HDL levels. When all else fails, certain drugs can effectively treat high cholesterol. Your physician will be able to advise you on whether drug treatment would be appropriate in your case.

Maintain A Varied Diet

All dietary experts generally recommend a varied diet of nutritious foods. This used to mean that we should include portions from the "four basic food groups," meat, dairy, grains, and fruits and vegetables, in our daily diet. The four food groups have since been supplanted by the food pyramid in the U.S. Department of Agriculture's updated dietary guidelines. Breads, cereals, pasta and grains serve as the foundation of the pyramid — six servings a day, including several servings of whole-grain products daily. Two servings of fruit and three servings of vegetables per day are also recommended. Meat, poultry, fish, and other protein sources, merit only two servings every day. Recommended daily consumption of dairy sources is likewise a mere two servings per day in a healthy diet .

The new guidelines are an outgrowth of research that shows the foundation of a healthy diet should be whole grains, fruits and vegetables. On the other hand, the role of the meat and dairy groups, once seen as staples of a nutritious diet, are significantly diminished. The USDA also strongly advises limiting the consumption of fats, sweets, and alcoholic beverages.

Those contemplating or currently practicing vegetarianism should not interpret the reduced significance of meat and dairy in the new dietary recommendations as sufficient grounds for eliminating these food groups entirely from one's diet. Without proper care, a vegetarian diet may supply inadequate levels of essential amino acids, and could lead to nutritional deficiencies, such as a deficiency of zinc, a mineral central to prostate function (*see p. 139*). However, with proper planning, a varied vegetarian diet can supply all the essential nutrients.

This points up the importance of practicing variety within food groups as well. A diet in which vegetable content is supplied only by corn and potatoes will be deficient in many essential nutrients. In fact, scientists are only beginning to learn how important variety is to a healthy diet. The recent discovery of *phytochemicals,* naturally produced chemicals in plants that possess an apparent ability to block carcinogenic processes (*see p. 137*), indicates that the well-established vitamins and minerals are not the only compounds found in plants that provide health benefits. Frequent rotation of foods, especially whole foods, is one way to ensure a varied, nutritious diet.

Eat Cancer-Fighting Foods

While a healthy diet ought to provide all the nutrients needed by the body, research indicates that certain vitamins, minerals, and chemicals found in foods are particularly useful in combating cancer. These natural substances use a number of mechanisms to protect the body from cancer formation and proliferation. The following may be of use in the fight against prostate cancer:

• *Vitamin D.* Epidemiological studies, which track broad patterns of diet and disease in the population, indicate that vitamin D may help prevent prostate cancer. In fact, several recent studies indicate that exposure to sunlight can significantly reduce the risk of prostate cancer, presumably due to the skin's conversion of sunlight into vitamin D. Besides sunlight, the best sources for this vitamin are sardines, fortified milk, and egg yolks.

• *Antioxidants.* This group of nutrients include vitamins A, C, E, selenium and beta-carotene, which is converted into vitamin A by the body. They are all the rage these days — in the popular media and with health-conscious consumers. And for good reason. Antioxidants are reputed by many to be a panacea for the great medical ills of our times. Indeed, although slow in coming, scientific evidence is accumulating that these substances provide protection against such deadly disorders as heart disease and cancer.

Current theory holds that antioxidants work to block the formation in the body of dangerous forms of oxygen known as *free radicals*. These free radicals are believed to damage cell membranes, and thus compromise the ability of a cell to perform essential tasks, such as the control of metabolism, regeneration of internal damage, and expulsion of bacteria, viruses, and toxins from the cell. If this theory is correct, antioxidant vitamins may short-circuit processes that lead to cancer.

Up to this point, the data has been inconclusive. The latest findings have certainly shown that antioxidants are not the "magic pill" against cancer that some have hoped. Large-scale studies are currently underway to better judge the health benefits of these substances.

In the meantime, there is no reason you should stand on the sidelines and wait while science makes up its mind. As they say, the best defense is a good offense. Take action by including foods rich in antioxidants in your diet. In its active form, vitamin A is found only in animal products such as whole milk, eggs, and meat, especially liver. Because many of these foods should be eaten only in moderation, it is probably better to rely on the vitamin A precursor, beta-carotene, for this valuable nutrient. It is found in a wide range of green and yellow fruits and vegetables. Orange juice, as well as tomatoes, broccoli, Brussels sprouts, cabbage, green peppers, and spinach, are good sources of vitamin C. Foods rich in vitamin E include green leafy vegetables, whole grains, and vegetable oils.

Selenium works in conjunction with vitamin E, and is found in meat, seafood, and whole grains.

Overcooking food can eliminate important nutrients, and because many vitamins are water-soluble, they can be lost through boiling. To avoid the loss of valuable nutrients, it is best to eat fruits and vegetables raw or steamed. Those concerned that their diet is not supplying sufficient quantities of these important nutrients can supplement their diet with a multivitamin. Further supplementation should be undertaken with caution. Reliance on the use of vitamin and mineral supplements remains controversial, especially when taken in doses far exceeding the recommended daily allowances (RDA), a practice known as *megadosing.* Megadoses of certain vitamins and minerals can be harmful, even fatal. No one should attempt self-treatment using vitamin and mineral supplements without first consulting his physician. For more on this subject, *see Nutritional Supplements,* beginning on p. 141.

• *Phytochemicals.* Until just a few years ago, no one even knew of the existence of phytochemicals. Out of this surprise discovery came a further revelation. Early experiments indicate that these mysterious biochemicals may turn out to be powerful new allies in the war on cancer!

Phytochemicals are naturally occurring chemicals found in plants ("phyto" is derived from the Greek word for plant), apparently serving to protect plants from the harmful effects of sunlight. Amazingly, medical researchers are uncovering hard evidence that they serve a completely different function as cancer-fighting agents in the human body. A myriad of these biochemicals exist in the fruits and vegetables we eat — it's been estimated that there are 10,000 in tomatoes alone! Although they have yet to draw the media blitz generated by antioxidants (that will come soon enough), phytochemicals have caught the immediate attention of both private and public institutions in the health industry. The National Cancer Institute itself has already launched a multimillion-dollar project to isolate and study them.

Experimental evidence has been plentiful to show the microscopic activities of these chemicals in slowing or reversing the mechanisms that lead to the growth of malignant tumors. *P-coumaric acid* and *chlorogenic acid,* found in tomatoes as well as several other fruits and vegetables, block the formation of carcinogenic compounds called nitrosomes. A phytochemical in turnips eliminates enzymes that cause cellular mutations. *Sulforaphane,* just one of many phytochemicals found in broccoli, retards the development of breast tumors in mice. Laboratory experiments indicate the phytochemical works by synthesizing enzymes which attach to carcinogenic molecules and drag them out of the cells before any damage can be done. Citrus fruits, berries, and a number of vegetables contain *flavanoids,* phytochemicals that keep cancer-causing hormones from fastening onto cells. These chemicals might be advantageous to prostate cancer patients, since most cases of prostate cancer are hormone-dependent.

The most significant find for men with prostate cancer is a chemical in soybeans called *genistein*, recently discovered by German researchers. Genistein acts to prevent the formation of capillaries around a malignant tumor, essentially cutting off the tumor's supply lines, and halting its growth. This finding has prompted researchers to suggest that the cause for the elevated risk of prostate cancer among Asian men who emigrate to the U.S. may be due to the adoption of a soy-poor American diet.

Investigation of phytochemicals is in its infancy. Although synthetic versions of sulforaphane have been created in the laboratory, in all likelihood it will be many years before you'll be able to get your phytochemicals in a pill. Until then, make sure you eat plenty of whole fruits and vegetables. Another pleasant surprise, most of the phytochemicals mentioned above seem to hold up fine through a variety of cooking processes.

• *Zinc*. The prostate gland contains higher concentrations of zinc than any other part of the body. The exact relationship between zinc and the prostate is unknown, but there is evidence that a zinc deficiency might precede the development of prostate problems, including prostate cancer. For this reason, eating foods containing zinc may be helpful. Foods rich in zinc include pumpkin seeds, oysters and other seafood, nuts, wheat bran and wheat germ, milk, eggs, onions, poultry, gelatin, beans, peas, lentils, and beef liver. Overcooking will deplete the natural zinc content of most foods.

Zinc supplements are sometimes prescribed to treat the symptoms of prostate enlargement and prostatitis, and should only be taken under the supervision of a physician. Excluding instances in which a zinc deficiency exists, there is no solid evidence that zinc supplements are effective in treating prostate cancer.

Avoid Cancer-Promoting Agents

While you are taking the necessary steps to ensure you eat a diet rich in cancer-inhibiting nutrients, do yourself a favor and do away with those substances that have been shown to contribute to cancer.

First among these is tobacco, which has been convincingly linked to the development of a number of cancers. Although many studies have shown that beta-carotene intake reduces the risk of lung cancer, a recent Finnish study showed no reduction in the incidence of lung cancer or any other cancer from the intake of carotenoid vitamin A or other antioxidants among heavy smokers. Apparently, antioxidants are no match for the devastating impact of cigarette smoking. Smoking also weakens the immune system. Now is the time to end this unhealthy habit.

Alcohol has been implicated as a cancer-promoting substance as well. It is also a prostate irritant. Try to limit your consumption of alcohol, or better yet, eliminate it from your life altogether.

Smoked foods and charbroiled, blackened, or overcooked meats are particularly high in carcinogens. Do your best to avoid them.

Nutritional Supplements

Vitamins are natural substances that have been scientifically established to be essential for physical health and life. A deficiency in any of the essential vitamins will result in serious health problems, a painful truth learned from such deadly maladies as scurvy and rickets (the consequence of deficiencies of vitamins C and D respectively). The development of natural and synthetic vitamin supplements was aimed at the prevention of such deficiencies. Now most deficiencies can be prevented or corrected through the use of supplements.

And yet the value of certain vitamin and mineral supplements — the antioxidants, vitamins A, C, E, and selenium — has become a subject of heated debate over the past decade. Central to the debate is not whether they have nutritional value and are able to prevent deficiency disorders, but if they have therapeutic value. Specifically at issue: are large doses, or *megadoses,* of these nutritional supplements of any benefit in the medical treatment or prevention of diseases such as cancer?

Governmental agencies, particularly the Food and Drug Administration (FDA), strongly oppose the promotion of unproved claims about the health benefits of these nutritional supplements.

Currently, FDA regulations do not permit unsubstantiated claims to appear on the labels of nutritional supplements concerning their capacity to prevent cancer, heart disease, or other diseases. The use of folic acid to prevent birth defects and calcium to prevent osteoporosis are the only exceptions, given that there is "significant scientific agreement among qualified experts" that these claims are valid. Conservative nutritionists side with the government, believing that megadosing is an expensive and potentially hazardous health fad, driven by profit.

Proponents of the medicinal use of vitamin and mineral megadosages argue that, even though scientific confirmation is not yet in, the American public should not be denied information on a potentially lifesaving alternative. They cite numerous studies documenting the cancer-preventing powers of nutritional supplements (much as their opponents cite studies that fail to show any positive effects from vitamin megadoses). When it comes to the health benefits of nutritional supplements in excess of the recommended daily allowances (RDAs), the opinions of physicians and other health professionals vary widely. Many conventional physicians question the value of using vitamin megadoses as a form of therapy, but consider the practice largely harmless if proper precautions are taken. In the meantime, the commercial marketing of vitamin and mineral supplements has become a multibillion dollar industry.

No doubt debate will continue, and this appendix certainly does not aim to resolve this dispute.

However, for those who are interested in exploring this avenue of self-treatment, information on specific antioxidants promoted by some as useful for men with prostate cancer is given below.

Vitamin A (Retinol) and Beta–Carotene

All of the retinoid vitamin A in our diets comes from animal sources. Beta-carotene on the other hand is found only in fruits and vegetables, and is known as a "dimer" of vitamin A, essentially two vitamin A molecules linked together. The liver acts to convert beta-carotene into active vitamin A.

Both animal studies and observational trials with humans have demonstrated a connection between low levels of these nutrients in the diet and increased risk of a variety of cancers. Early anticancer studies focused on vitamin A, but the evidence to date points to beta-carotene as a better antioxidant and more effective anticancer agent. It has been suggested that the antioxidant characteristics of beta-carotene supplementation can be particularly effective in preventing the recurrence of cancer tumors following treatment.

High doses of retinoid vitamin A taken daily for a prolonged period can cause harmful, even fatal, liver damage. Therefore, supplementation with beta-carotene is generally preferred. Excessive dosages of beta-carotene may cause a yellowing of the skin, called carotenosis, but this condition is apparently harmless.

The recommended daily allowance (RDA) for vitamin A is 5,000 IU (international units). Those who advocate the therapeutic use of beta-carotene megadoses typically advise a daily dosage ten, twenty, or even thirty times the RDA for good nutrition. It is worth noting that vitamin A in the bloodstream has been found to be significantly lower in prostate cancer patients than in other men, although the reason for this is unclear. As a cautionary note, it has been suggested that increased vitamin A consumption over several years could lead to a chronic lowering of zinc levels within the prostate, a condition that some believe to be a factor in the early growth of prostate cancer.

Vitamin C (Ascorbic Acid)

Nobel Laureate Dr. Linus Pauling, who popularized the use of vitamin C as a remedy for the common cold, has also been a vocal advocate for the use of vitamin C supplements in the prevention and treatment of cancer. Vitamin C is not only a powerful antioxidant, but plays an important role in the proper functioning of the immune system. During the seventies, Pauling conducted several studies that showed high doses of supplemental vitamin C increased survival time and improved the quality of life among terminal cancer patients. Three randomized trials by the National Cancer Institute failed to confirm Dr. Pauling's findings, although Dr. Pauling has strongly criticized the manner in which these studies were conducted. Subsequent studies have overall been inconclusive.

Undaunted, Dr. Pauling continues to preach the virtues of vitamin C. In 1992, he claimed vitamin C is effective in reducing prostate tumors. Although Pauling's views may yet be vindicated, the jury is still out on the effectiveness of vitamin C supplements as a useful therapy for cancer.

The RDA for vitamin C is 60 milligrams, but the vitamin is generally considered non-toxic at much higher dosages. The most common side effect of excessive vitamin C is diarrhea. Rare complications have been known to result as a consequence of megadosing. Also, the body becomes conditioned to higher intake of vitamin C, and abrupt cessation of a high dosage could result in a dangerous drop of vitamin C in the blood. Dosages far in excess of nutritional needs should not be taken without the consent and oversight of a physician.

Vitamin E (Tocopherol)

This antioxidant vitamin has been the subject of much attention of late. Most of this interest revolves around recent evidence that megadoses of vitamin E ten to twenty times the RDA of 30 IU may help to prevent heart attacks. Two Harvard studies, published in the New England Journal of Medicine (May 20, 1993) tracked 87,000 female and

40,000 male health care professionals over a span of several years. The studies report that up to 40% reduction in risk of heart attacks was seen among men and women on a daily dose of vitamin E ranging from 100 to 250 IU. No additional benefit could be detected at higher doses.

This is perhaps the closest thing to confirmation yet seen that vitamins in megadose quantities may have a medicinal use beyond the vitamin's established nutritional function. Yet even so, the medical community remains skeptical. The American Heart Association refuses to recommend vitamin E supplements "until more complete data are available."

Vitamin E is believed to possess anti-aging properties, and in significant quantities appears to stimulate the immune system. Use of vitamin E supplements for the prevention of certain cancers has been quite promising, but to date inconclusive. Like vitamins A and D, vitamin E is a fat-soluble vitamin and will collect in the body. However, vitamin E seems to be much safer than A and D in large doses. Still, researchers caution that the safety of vitamin E megadoses taken over an extended period have not been established by rigorous scientific testing.

Vitamin E works synergistically with selenium in the body, and taking them in conjunction enhances their beneficial properties.

Selenium

An essential trace mineral, selenium is needed by the body for pancreatic function and to maintain tissue elasticity. Selenium is also a broad-spectrum antioxidant. It has been well-established that selenium and vitamin E work together to aid in production of antibodies. Animal studies have found selenium retards tumor formation. One of these studies also noted that ending selenium supplementation in animals resulted in a sudden increase in tumor development. Those who advocate taking selenium to prevent cancer caution against sudden cessation of supplementation.

Studies have found regions rich in selenium correlate with lower incidence of cancer in the population, including prostate cancer. As with vitamins A, C, and E, several studies have found that individuals with low serum (blood) selenium levels had a significantly higher risk of developing cancer. Experimentation indicates that some cancer patients have difficulty absorbing selenium when taken as oral supplements. A large-scale NCI study is currently underway to investigate the effects of selenium supplementation.

The RDA for selenium is 70 micrograms, but it has been argued that only megadose quantities in the several hundreds of micrograms or even higher can successfully increase blood levels of selenium. Caution should be practiced in taking large doses of selenium, since the mineral can be quite toxic. Bad breath is one harmless side-effect of selenium megadoses, but more severe symptoms result as a consequence of selenium toxicity, such as extreme nausea and weakness, with accompanying discoloration of the fingernails. Close medical supervision and testing of blood selenium levels is necessary to prevent toxicity in those taking large doses of this mineral.

Supplemental Suggestions

Whether you should take nutritional supplements is up to you. The safest route — and one recommended by the FDA — is to get your antioxidants in the foods you eat every day.

You may wish to take more aggressive action. One thing you could do is get a blood test. If you have low levels of key nutrients in your bloodstream, you may be more likely to benefit from supplements. But keep in mind that megadosages can be hazardous, and some supplements may interact with various medications or pose a health risk for men with medical conditions other than prostate cancer. Always seek the advice of a physician before beginning any vitamin regimen.

One additional point should be made. Although much has been made of studies indicating the promise of antioxidants as cancer-fighting agents, nutritional supplements are no substitute for a good diet and a healthy lifestyle. Don't make them a substitute for practicing healthy habits in your life.

Chapter 10

THE HEALING SEED

"*Two roads diverged in a wood, and I—*
I took the one less traveled by,
And that has made all the difference."

Robert Frost

Months had passed since my fateful discovery that I had prostate cancer.

Meanwhile, winter had changed to spring, and soon, spring would succomb to summer. The gray skies and chill winds of February, when I first learned of my cancer, had given way to spring rains, green grass and blooming flowers. Everywhere, lizards scampered in the bright sunlight, and down by the water's edge, trains of ducklings waddled single-file after their mothers. The season had brought its recurrent gift of new life, light, and hope.

But little had changed for me.

I had returned from the fog-shrouded city of Baltimore with a date for my operation at Johns Hopkins Hospital on August 6th. I had hoped for something more —— or less; something intangible. Peace, clarity, resolution. What I really longed for was a sense of conclusion to the dilemma of the past several months.

And yet in the days that followed, as I once again returned to work at my law practice, there remained a lingering uncertainty. Niggling doubts about whether I was doing the right thing, if there might have been something I had missed. Everything I had been told, everything I had learned, pushed me toward my present path. The way seemed clear, yet after all these months, something within me still resisted traveling the road laid out for me. Within my mind, one thought repeatedly asserted itself. Was a radical prostatectomy operation really the best course for me, or might there still be another, better way?

The Road Less Traveled

At some point in my readings, I had come across the number for the National Cancer Institute's hotline, 1-800-4-CANCER. I had tried the number on many occasions, with no success. Each time, I had gotten a busy signal. It was an indication for me of just how many people there were out there struggling with a disease like mine, searching for answers.

Finally, about the middle of May, I got through. I talked to a woman named Maria. The first thing she asked me to do was to read to her the results of my biopsy and subsequent staging tests. I had been clinically diagnosed with stage B2 prostate cancer, the latest stage of prostate cancer still confined to the prostate. It was still curable, but only if I acted in time.

I indicated that I was familiar with the conventional treatments for prostate cancer, but wanted to find out if there were any other options I could pursue.

Maria made it clear that she could not advise me concerning which treatment I selected, but she could tell me my alternatives. Then she asked me, given the stage of my cancer, what I understood my options to be.

I said, "It looks like I have three choices: I can have the radical prostatectomy, external radiation therapy, or I can do nothing — maybe not the wisest choice, but at least it is another option. I guess that's about it."

"No, Mr. Kaltenbach," she said, "You have a fourth choice."

"Oh?"

And then she told me about a new treatment: brachytherapy, using palladium seeds implanted directly into the prostate. At first, I was disappointed. I had heard about the use of radioactive seed implants before. From what I had been able to gather, major abdominal surgery was involved, and the results obtained with the treatment had never been particularly promising.

But this was something different. The procedure used was quite new, and was performed on an outpatient basis, without cutting. Significant improvements over previous seed implantation procedures made this treatment a real, viable alternative for someone with prostate cancer. Suddenly, I was very excited.

As Maria described it to me, tiny titanium tubes filled with the radioactive isotope palladium-103 are injected into the cancerous prostate. The seeds are visually guided into place with the use of ultrasound technology, ensuring that the implants are evenly apportioned throughout the prostate gland. Once planted, the radiation within the seeds goes to work, killing the cancer. Designed to irradiate only the site of the cancer, palladium seed implants can deliver a much higher dose of radiation than external beam radiation, with far fewer resulting complications.

The palladium implants, known as TheraSeeds, had only been in use for a few months, but possessed distinct advantages over alternative sources of radiation, such as the commonly-used iodine-125 seed implants. Palladium has a half-life of only 17 days, and degrades rapidly compared with the 60 day half-life of radioactive iodine. Within six months, or about 10 half-lives, the palladium seeds become inert, and reside harmlessly within the prostate.

Furthermore, the initial burst of radiation produced by palladium seeds is significantly higher, with lethal consequences for the cancer. Cancer tumors are destroyed rapidly, with no time to recover. And the effective range of radiation emitted by the palladium seeds is only about a centimeter, thus avoiding any threat of damage to surrounding organs.

At a time when I was floundering, this news was a godsend. I thanked Maria and immediately called Theragenics, the manufacturers of the TheraSeed implant, located in Norcross, Georgia. They informed me that at the time there were only two cancer centers in the country performing the palladium seed implant procedure. One was located in Seattle and headed by Dr. John Blasko. The other was the Georgia Prostate Center in Atlanta, founded and directed by Dr. Harold P. McDonald.

Over the next week, I spoke to Dr. McDonald on several occasions. He was friendly, but very professional. We discussed my condition at length, and he answered all of my questions with great patience. He also sent me a packet of information on the procedure.

I was very encouraged by everything I learned, but I wanted to be certain I made the right decision. As I began to develop a relationship with Dr. McDonald, I expressed to him my concerns.

"I need to find a comfort level with this procedure," I told him. "This is a new treatment, and I want to make sure I won't be some sort of test subject. Would you mind if I spoke to some of your patients?"

He gave me six names, and I called them all. Each man I talked to raved about the seed implant procedure. One was forty-one years old, about my own age. He encouraged me to have the procedure done as soon as possible. Only one of the men had experienced any difficulties after being treated ---- he had gone square dancing the weekend following his operation. Afterwards, he had been very sore, and temporarily had a catheter put in. But what really amazed me was that he had felt well enough a couple days after an operation to go square dancing in the first place! It was a testimony to the ease of recovery following this treatment.

The enthusiasm of these men for the procedure was infectious. As I listened to their stories, they described their struggle with the same concerns that I was now experiencing: the desire to avoid the costs and dangers of major surgery, the fear of impotency and incontinence that often resulted from the conventional treatments, the hope for some better alternative. For them, the answer had been palladium seed implantation. I was beginning to believe it was the answer for me as well.

With growing confidence, I called the McDonald clinic to find out what arrangements were necessary if I chose to have the procedure done. I talked with one of the nurses on McDonald's staff, providing her with biographical information — details on my medical history, my insurance coverage, and the like. While I was talking with her, I made a surprising discovery. Nine years earlier, she had lived in New Port Richey and had been a client of mine! In fact, she had actually worked for the local urologist who had diagnosed my prostate cancer. It was a coincidence that seemed almost providential.

There was really no point in delaying any longer. I knew this was the right choice for me. I called Johns Hopkins and, with some relief, canceled my operation. Then I got back with the McDonald clinic and set a date for the seed implantation. When I hung up the phone, a feeling washed over me that seemed almost unfamiliar, given the turmoil of the recent months. It was peace of mind.

In and Out By Lunchtime

The day before the operation, Nancy and I flew up to Georgia. I needed a battery of tests done the night before. It was all rather routine. By now I was an old hand at test-taking.

The preoperative ultrasound and CT scan were particularly important. They are used to calculate the volume and position of the prostate in the body, an essential element of the preplanning stage of the procedure. The data generated is

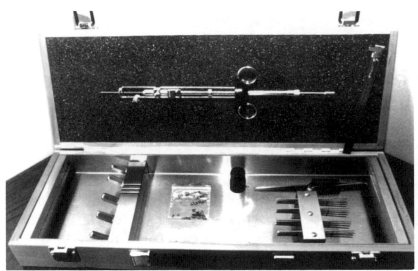

Courtesy of Theragenics, Inc.

Figure 12. Hollow needles (stylets) and device for implanting radioactive seeds.

analyzed using a computer to determine the optimal dose of radiation and proper distribution of the palladium seeds. The precise and specialized preparation involved in this procedure results in a treatment plan individualized to the patient. The number of seeds implanted, the number of implant needles used, and the configuration used in the placement of the seeds all vary according to the needs of the specific patient. This careful planning ensures that the ideal level of radiation is administered to all areas of the patient's prostate.

The template and implant needles were prepared the night before my operation, based on my individualized treatment plan. To prepare for the procedure, the palladium seeds, which look like little pieces of pencil lead, are inserted into the implant needles. An implant needle consists of a pointed stylet within a sleeve. Once the stylet is withdrawn, the seeds are dropped into the hollow tube of the sleeve, each seed one half centimeter apart. The number of seeds per needle vary from two to five. Each needle is numbered depending on the hole in the template into which it is to be inserted. The template itself is a square Lexan plate. The holes in this plate guide the needles as they are inserted into the prostate gland, where the seeds are then deposited.

I was admitted into the medical center a couple hours prior to undergoing the procedure. Three other men were to receive palladium seed implantation that same morning. I was to be the last.

Since the procedure was non-invasive, meaning no incision was to be made, I was given the option of receiving local or general anesthesia. I chose the local anesthetic, since it would give me the opportunity to talk on the intercom with Nancy, who would be watching the operation on a TV monitor in an observation room.

When my time came, I was wheeled over to the OR and placed on an operating table in what they call the "semilithotomy position," a fancy name meaning you are on your back with your legs in stirrups. I guess it doesn't sound nearly so degrading put that way! Naturally, the staff was very professional, although I do recall a couple of jokes in the OR about how it was "nice to see a man in stirrups for a change" — an attitude no doubt endorsed by many women, including my wife.

Once on the table, I was prepped for the procedure. I was injected with the local anesthetic, and the template was put in place up flush with the perineum, the region directly between the legs. Cloth was draped over me, to provide me with some measure of privacy.

An abdominal catheter was put in place, to drain urine from the bladder during the operation. Then Dr. McDonald performed the seed implantation. Each needle was inserted into the prostate to a depth previously determined by the computerized treatment plan, and the sleeve of the needle withdrawn, leaving the seeds implanted within the prostate. Once in place, the tiny seeds appeared as rows of white dashes on the ultrasound monitor. Sixty-three seeds later, it was all over. The entire operation was completed in under an hour.

About one o'clock, I was wheeled into a lounge. The anesthetic hadn't worn off, and so my legs weren't working yet. There, Nancy and I met with the three other men who underwent the operation that morning and their wives. At Dr. McDonald's suggestion, we had all brought sack lunches. So we sat and ate our lunches, and talked about the procedure. The always jovial Dr. McDonald dropped in on us to chat for a few minutes before getting back to work.

A few hours later, I walked out of the Georgia Prostate Center into the bright Antlanta sunlight, carrying with me sixty-three radioactive seeds silently at work destroying my cancer. It boggled my mind to think that, but for a single phone call a couple of weeks earlier, I would have at this point endured major abdominal surgery and all its inherent risks. With the radical prostatectomy, I

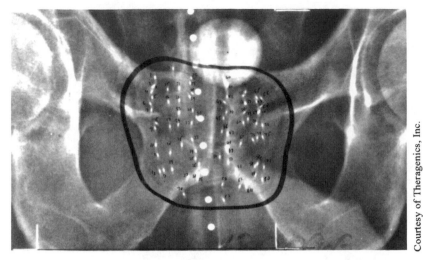

Figure 13. An x-ray of the prostate following brachytherapy. As shown in the photo, the seeds are carefully numbered and accounted for as part of the follow-up procedure.

would have had a five to ten day hospital stay, followed by at least six weeks of bed rest. But instead, after a routine check-up the next morning, I would be on my way home, and within a couple of days I could safely return to work. The long-term picture also looked good: unlike the surgical option, the likelihood of significant complications with the seed implantation treatment was small. I couldn't help but feel lucky.

The weekend after the operation, I was hiking with my kids in the mountains of North Carolina. Although it was now the second week of June, to me it seemed that spring had finally arrived.

Chapter 11

LIFE AFTER
PROSTATE CANCER

"Timely wise accept the terms,
Soften the fall with wary foot;
A little while
Still plan and smile..."

Ralph Waldo Emerson

Three months after my treatment for prostate cancer, I returned to the McDonald clinic for my quarterly check-up. I was glad to see the friendly faces of Dr. McDonald and his staff. They had become like family to me.

I was also anxious to find out if the treatment had worked. They gave me a PSA test to measure the level of prostate specific antigen in my bloodstream, followed by an ultrasound of the prostate itself. The blood test indicated my PSA level had dropped to 1.3, well within the normal range.

And the tumor in my prostate no longer showed up on ultrasound.

To all appearances, I was cancer-free.

Only someone who has gone through treatment for cancer can imagine the relief I felt at this good news. The cancer was gone!

The journey was finally over, I said to myself. It seemed as though I had passed through some unknown land, lost and trying to find my way. With searching and setbacks, twisting roads and dangerous obstacles, I had finally made it to my destination. I was cured. Now life could return to normal again.

Or so I thought.

"So when do I get my certificate declaring I am officially cured?" I asked Dr. McDonald.

"I'm afraid I can't give you one of those." he said apologetically. "You're in remission now, but we can't guarantee the cancer won't return sometime in the future."

This was not the news I was hoping for. The realization that I would never be, with absolute certainty, cured of cancer was a hard blow to take. I wanted it to be all over. I wanted to drop the whole mess in the "Out" basket and have it all go away. Unfortunately, with cancer, that isn't the way it works. All I could do was watch and wait. And hope for the best.

With every passing year, the chances increase that the cancer will not return. Every quarter, I have more tests to check my progress. So far, after more than four years, I remain free of cancer.

Coping With Complications

I was one of the lucky ones. I have gotten through the ordeal of prostate cancer largely unscathed. Many men are not so fortunate. Even men who are successfully treated may find their victory over prostate cancer eclipsed by subsequent side effects of their treatment. Just when the battle appears to be over, they find themselves in a new struggle. For some men, the complications associated with a potential cure seem worse than the disease itself.

The most common and distressing of these complications are impotence and incontinence. Yet medical science can help those men who suffer from these side-effects. In almost every case, some treatment is available to improve the quality of life of those struggling to cope with impotence or incontinence.

Impotence

Impotence is defined as the consistent inability to achieve or sustain an erection sufficient for sexual intercourse. It is also referred to by doctors as erectile dysfunction.

Until recently, the vast majority of men became impotent following a radical prostatectomy.

The new nerve-sparing technique pioneered by Dr. John Walsh of Johns Hopkins now preserves potency in many cases. However, even with this procedure, sexual function may be temporarily or permanently lost. Temporary impotence may last up to twelve months after surgery. When the problem persists beyond this length of time, the damage is often permanent.

Impotence may result from other common treatments for prostate cancer as well. Most men retain potency following radiation therapy, but may develop an impotence problem a year or two following treatment. Impotence is also a common consequence of an orchiectomy and the use of hormonal therapy to treat prostate cancer.

Some men who are in their later years and no longer sexually active suffer little impact from this complication. However, most of those who were still sexually active at treatment will be anxious to take some action to restore their loss of ability to achieve an erection.

There is no simple test for impotence. The only way a doctor knows that an impotence problem exists is through the statement of the patient himself. To complicate matters, impotence may have both psychological or physical roots, and in some cases both play a role in an impotency problem. Sometimes merely anticipating that they will be impotent after treatment will cause men to experience a loss of function. Stress, anxiety and depression can also effect sexual function.

A diagnostic analysis will be the first step in treating impotence. This will begin with a period of detailed questioning to clarify the nature of the problem. One thing the doctor will try to learn is if the ability to attain erection varies depending on the time or circumstances. If so, at least part of the problem is psychological and may be treated through counseling.

To ascertain if there is a medical basis for the problem, the doctor will usually perform certain tests. These may include measurements of blood pressure and pulse in the penis to locate circulation problems that might be responsible for erectile dysfunction. A blood test may be used to check the level of male hormones. Because men experience erections during sleep, a sleep laboratory evaluation may also be performed. A simple and inexpensive version of this test can be performed by the patient himself at home. Normal erections experienced during sleep indicate that the impotence problem does not have a physical basis.

In many cases, however, a physical cause for the impotence problem will be found. There are several potential physical causes of impotence. Both surgery and radiation therapy can damage the nerves that control erection. Vascular damage is another common cause of physical impotence after treatment for prostate cancer, and results in a reduction of blood flow to the penis needed to achieve and sustain an erection. Hormones are involved in the ability to attain an erection as well. Hormonal therapy, which blocks the production of testosterone, the primary male sex hormone, often results in a loss of sexual desire and erection problems. Certain medications, such as those used to treat high blood pressure and depression, may produce impotence as well.

There are a variety of treatments available for men suffering from impotence. These include the following:

• *Injections.* A variety of drugs can be used in the treatment of impotence. Papaverine, Regatine (phentolamine mesylate), and prostaglandin are the most common drugs used to relax muscles and increase the blood supplied to the penis. Injections are made directly into the penis, initially by the physician and later by the patient himself. Although many men find the idea of penile injections unpleasant, they cause only minimal discomfort. Men uncomfortable with needles can get a simple device that automatically injects medication with the press of a button. Research is currently underway to develop a drug patch or preparation that can be applied externally, eliminating the need for injections altogether.

For many men, these injections will prove very effective in restoring lost function, but for those who have had extensive damage to the blood vessels in the vicinity of the prostate, due to surgery or radiation therapy, injections may produce unsatisfactory results.

• *Penile Implants.* Intrapenile prosthetic devices can be a satisfactory solution for men who wish to continue having intercourse. The penile prosthesis is placed inside the corpora cavernosa, two tube-like structures within the penis that fill with blood to produce erection. The many penile implants currently available fall into two basic categories: those that are inflatable and those that are semi-rigid. The advantages and disadvantages of each type of prosthesis should be discussed between the patient and his physician. Men should also be sure to include their partner in any decision about implants.

• *Vacuum Devices.* These non-surgical devices use vacuum suction and penile constriction to assist blood flow into the penis, causing an erection. They consist of a plastic cylinder placed over the penis and a hand-held pump to draw air from the cylinder. Once erection is achieved, an elastic band is placed around the base of the penis to maintain erection. Although less popular than injections or implant devices, these devices have the advantage of being non-invasive. Many men report successful use of vacuum-constriction devices.

• *Surgical Treatment.* For those who suffer from vascular blockage, an experimental surgical procedure can be performed. An artery that usually supplies blood to the stomach is rerouted by the surgeon and connected to blood vessels inside the penis. So far, the results have been somewhat disappointing.

These treatments enable many men with erectile dysfunction to enjoy normal sexual relations. However, one should be realistic about what these methods can and cannot do. Those who suffer from low sexual desire or decreased sensation may not be entirely satisfied with the results that these treatments provide.

Beyond these treatments for physical impotence, certain changes can be made to counteract factors that may be contributing to the sexual impairment. Medications that contribute to an impotence problem or a loss of sexual desire can often be exchanged for others that do not have these side effects. Other complications, such as pain or fatigue, may also be contributing factors. Treating these conditions may help. Lifestyle changes, such as improved diet, exercise, and reduced consumption of alcohol, can also lead to improved sexual performance. When psychological or emotional issues are involved, sex therapy or counseling often serve to decrease performance anxiety and reduce mental blocks to satisfying sex. See also *Overcoming the Threat to Intimacy, on p. 171.*

Incontinence

Urinary incontinence — the involuntary loss of bladder control — is caused by damage to the bladder neck, external urethral sphincter, or musculature surrounding the prostate gland, and may result from the use of any of the surgical techniques involved in the treatment of prostate cancer. The condition may last weeks, months, or for more prolonged periods of time.

The most common form is referred to as *stress incontinence,* a relatively mild condition that involves the involuntry leakage of urine at moments of increased pressure on the bladder, such as can occur from coughing, sneezing, or heavy lifting. *Urgency incontinence,* exemplified by an inability to delay urination when the bladder feels full, may sometimes result from treatment of prostate cancer as well. In rare cases, severe incontinence may occur, resulting in a complete loss of ability to retain urine.

Many effective treatments for incontinence exist. After a patient reports a problem with urinary control, the urologist performs an evaluation to determine the nature and extent of the incontinence. Depending on the results of this evaluation, the doctor will recommend an appropriate treatment option or options. Some of the treatments available include:

• *Medications.* If only partial damage has been sustained by the muscles controlling retention of urine, various drugs, such as Ephedrine, can be used to contract remaining muscle tissue. This treatment can restore or improve continence in many cases. Drug treatment may also be used to relax the bladder and reduce the pressure it exerts on stored urine, thus minimizing leakage.

• *Kegel exercises.* Special exercises are another technique used to treat incontinence. Kegel exercises involve alternate tightening and relaxing of muscles at the base of the pelvis. Frequent use of Kegel exercises help to restore lost control in many men. Biofeedback is another means that may be used to train and strengthen the muscles that control urination.

• *Injections.* The use of collagen injections has received much attention of late. Collagen is found in the connective tissues that make up the joints and bones of animals and humans. Purified into a white, fibrous paste, collagen is injected into the neck of the bladder to narrow the urethral opening. Men whose urethral sphincter has been damaged by surgery may be good candidates for this treatment. The procedure used to inject the collagen takes about 30 minutes and is relatively inexpensive.

• *Artificial Sphincters.* If drug therapy and physical therapy are unsuccessful, and the patient is a poor candidate for collagen injections, then surgical means can be undertaken to treat incontinence as well. An artifical sphincter may be put in place to control urine flow. An inflatable circular cuff is put around the urethra, usually just below the external urethral sphincter. Once inflated, the flow of urine is cut off. When the need to void is felt, a pump mechanism can be triggered that will deflate the cuff, allowing urine to flow out of the bladder. After a brief period of time, the cuff will automatically reinflate. Even in the most severe cases of incontinence, these artificial sphincters can often dramatically improve the condition of the patient.

Even in cases where no cure is found, there are still several means to make an incontinence problem manageable and enable men to live a normal lifestyle. Developing a regular schedule for drinking and voiding can reduce many problems associated with incontinence. For overweight individuals, weight loss can significantly improve control by reducing pressure on the bladder. Avoidance of diuretic foods and drugs will also promote continence.

There are numerous absorbent products and devices that are comfortable and provide the individual with the freedom to remain active, regardless of the degree of incontinence. These range from drip collectors that fit over the penis to condom catheters that may be worn with a leg bag to collect urine.

It is an unfortunate fact that incontinence is a consequence of treatment for prostate cancer in a small percentage of men. But although incontinence is inconvenient and even unpleasant at times, with care and planning, no embarassment need ever result. With the extensive range of treatments and products now available, any man can learn to live his life without having to withdraw from society or give up any of the activities he enjoys.

Overcoming The Threat To Intimacy

For the majority of men with prostate cancer, following the threat to life itself, the threat to sexual intimacy is the greatest concern. Fortunately, there is no reason to assume that treatment for prostate cancer will end a man's sex life.

However, it is true that prostate cancer and the complications of treatment can affect a man's sexual relations. More than a little courage and adaptability may be needed to overcome sexual difficulties should they develop. It is a sad fact that some men and their partners surrender in the face of these difficulties, and give up an active sexual relationship. Tragically, some even withdraw from physical closeness altogether.

Changes in appearance and sexual capacities can be terrifying. Many of these fears are greatly intensified by the sexual myths that men first encounter in their adolescent years. They are such myths as: A real man never fails to achieve erection. A real man is always ready and willing. A real man is rugged, strong and vigorous. Although probably no man has ever fully lived up to the ideal these myths express, when faced with a sexual problem, almost every man is tormented by such ingrained notions of masculinity.

It is in the interest of every man to abandon these outgrown myths, whether he is struggling with a sexual problem or not. For all of us, age undermines those physical attributes that our youth culture identifies with sexuality. But the process of aging is also an opportunity to understand and more fully appreciate the deeper personal qualities that enrich our intimate relationships. As the importance of the physical aspects wane, the emphasis we give to mental, emotional, and spiritual aspects of sexuality grows in response.

This isn't to say that physical changes have no significance. They do. But don't overestimate their importance. If you feel less attractive, remember that your wife married a person, not a body. Your body may have changed, but you are still the same person you always were.

Similarly, complications of treatment may be troublesome, but need not end your sex life. Hygeinic precautions may be necessary, but no degree of incontinence need bar a man from engaging in sexual activity. Men who suffer impotence problems after surgery still experience desire and can still feel all the sensations associated with sex, including orgasm. Although it may be very difficult to adjust to emotionally, impotence is essentially a mechanical problem, and does not really reflect on your manhood. As already mentioned, there are many available treatments for impotence. Don't let embarrassment and fear of rejection keep you from seeking a workable solution.

Men who are receiving hormonal therapy may suffer a significant loss of desire as well as impotency problems. This is because in some mysterious way, male hormones are intimately involved in sexual arousal. However, a minority of men undergoing this kind of therapy remain sexually active and continue to feel desire. These men prove the axiom that the brain is the most important sex organ. Although the urge may have diminished, many more men might be capable of remaining sexually active if they learned how to encourage the more subtle sexual feelings that the mind can create.

Reinitiating sexual involvement with your partner involves a risk, especially when a sexual problem exists. It may help, in overcoming any feelings of inadequacy you may have, to better understand your partner's feelings about the matter. Many men have misconceptions about their spouse's sexual needs and desires. This issue became the topic of discussion at a recent Side by Side meeting, a support group sponsored by Man to Man for the wives of prostate cancer patients. During the meeting, one woman said, "I've loved my husband all my life. We've had a wonderful sexual relationship. I know what he's gone through, and I'm very content with being loved, having a lot of attention, having a special friend, hugging, kissing, and cuddling. We're doing more of that now, and I feel better than I did when we were able to have sexual intercourse."

Other women at the meeting expressed similar feelings, highlighting the importance of physical closeness and affection as an integral part of a woman's needs. A few years ago, Ann Landers conducted a survey of her female readership. It made the national news when the majority of the women who responded said they would dispense with sexual intercourse before they would give up physical closeness and affection with their mate. For most women, intercourse is clearly only one facet of sexual intimacy.

Before sexual expression can be reintroduced into your marriage, and sexual problems dealt with, you will need to talk openly with your wife. Communicating about this sensitive subject can be uncomfortable, but is really the only way to come to terms with the issue. Prolonging silence on the subject will only lead to a growing distance between you and your partner. And because most women are not sexual initiators, they usually find it at least as hard or harder than their husbands to broach the subject. Your wife may also be avoiding the issue of sex for fear of making you feel inadequate. Let her know you miss being intimate with her and would like to talk about ways of restoring your sex life.

Most therapists suggest gradually reintroducing sexual intimacy into your relationship. You might want to intentionally limit sexual expression to physical closeness and cuddling at first to help alleviate feelings of anxiety. Try to keep the atmosphere light and undemanding. This will enable both you and your partner to more easily come to terms with possible changes in your sexual relationship.

If you are simply unable to openly communicate with your partner about sex, or if you cannot overcome negative thoughts and feelings associated with a sexual problem, it may be appropriate to see a sex therapist. A qualified sex therapist is *not* a sex surrogate, but a health professional (a psychiatrist, social worker, or psychologist) who is trained in treating sexual problems. This typically involves discussion and "homework" assignments for the couple aimed at establishing better communication, reducing anxiety, and learning new sexual skills. There are also many self-help books available at libraries and bookstores that provide similar information. The booklet, *Sexuality and Cancer,* produced by the American Cancer Society, is also a valuable resource for men who wish to rekindle sexual expression after cancer treatment.

Keeping your sex life going in face of the obstacles that prostate cancer and its treatment often pose can be a challenge, but it is rewarding in the long run. Things may never be the same as they were before. Sex may not be spontaneous. Intercourse may be less frequent. Yet making the effort to restore your sexual relationship with your wife will give you the opportunity to find new means of intimate expression. Some couples may find that their physical relationship has been hindered by complications, but many of these couples discover a greater emotional intimacy in their marriage by striving to remain close. In a healthy relationship, there will always be ways of showing love and affection for each other. This is something that can never be taken from you.

The Conspiracy of Silence

Sometime after I had returned from my treatment by Dr. McDonald in Atlanta, I got a call from the local urologist who had diagnosed my cancer. He had advised me to have a radical prostatectomy and was curious to find out if I had had anything done for my prostate cancer.

I told him I had undergone palladium seed implantation.

"Oh, the McDonald clinic," he replied.

I hadn't mentioned the name of the clinic. It was clear that he had known about the procedure all along. Why hadn't he told me about it?

This incident stuck in my mind in the following months. I wondered how many other men were left in ignorance because their doctors failed in their duty to properly inform them of their options. It took me a while, but eventually I made my experience with prostate cancer public. I gave speeches at local group meetings in the hope of helping others. My message has been simple: men who turn 40 should have a prostate exam once a year; those who are diagnosed with prostate cancer need to take the steps to inform themselves about their options before taking action.

Since that time, rarely have I gone a day or two without receiving a call from someone with prostate cancer, or a friend or relative of a man with the disease. In many cases, my name came to them by word of mouth. They are often afraid and uncertain. Some of the men who call have just been diagnosed, and are terrified at what it might mean. I have listened to men in their seventies struggle to hold back tears as they tell me about their diagnosis with the disease. Some men have been told by their doctors to undergo a certain treatment and want a second opinion. Some have relapsed after treatment and want to know what to do now. One thing is common to all these men: they are desperate for information.

It never ceases to amaze me how little these men have been told. Most don't even know what stage of cancer they have. Nor are they usually familiar with their treatment options. Often, they have been left completely in the dark.

Lloyd Ney, founder of PAACT, a patient advocacy organization for prostate cancer, has called the failure of physicians to communicate the available options to the patient "the silent conspiracy." Many doctors are biased toward treatments provided by their specialty. A urologist will usually recommend surgery, a radiotherapist radiation therapy, or an oncologist hormonal treatment or chemotherapy. Specialists, aware of the widespread disagreement in the medical community concerning the best treatment for prostate cancer, may choose to shield their patients from the controversy. The price to the patient is the loss of his freedom to choose.

Some doctors are reticent to admit they are not fully informed about a particular disease, yet general practitioners may be unfamiliar with the latest and best treatments. No doubt there are some physicians who choose to keep their patients ignorant of alternatives for fear of losing revenue. Whatever the reason, doctors often fail to adequately tell their patients about their conditions and the treatments that are available. And all too often, patients are willing to relinquish their right to know the alternatives available to them in their longing to believe the doctor knows what is best for them.

Unfortunately, this unwillingness to fully disclose treatment options to the patient can lead to abuses. Anyone involved with cancer patients hears his share of horror stories. I myself have talked to men in their seventies with stage A prostate cancer who have been told they have no recourse but to get a radical prostatectomy. Yet in the majority of cases, stage A prostate cancer will never pose a threat to the life of the patient. This is especially true of older men, who will in all likelihood die of natural causes before the disease advances to a stage that poses a health risk. This kind of abuse is all too common, unfortunately. Two recent studies reported on in the Journal of the American Medical Association (May, 1993) indicate an increase in radical prostatectomy operations of 600% over the last six years, many of them unnecessary. One of the researchers commented, "When surgeons are in doubt, they cut." For men in their seventies and eighties with early stage prostate cancer, less aggressive treatment, or merely monitoring the progress of the disease, is usually a preferable approach.

On the other hand, there are those cases in which the physician treating a cancer patient inexplicably waits when more immediate treatment is appropriate. I remember one instance where a man in his sixties was diagnosed with early stage cancer and his doctor chose to simply monitor his PSA level. More than a year passed while his PSA steadily climbed, and his cancer progressed from its original B1 stage to stage D1. By that point, he had begun to experience symptoms of the disease. His chance for receiving curative treatment had been squandered.

Cases like these drove me to write this book, to help fill the void left by incommunicative physicians. As one who has experience as a prostate cancer patient, my hope is that this book might arm others like myself — who might otherwise be left without a full awareness of their alternatives — with the knowledge to ask the right questions of their physicians, and the necessary information to judge and evaluate the answers they receive.

Chapter 12

WHEN YOUR HUSBAND HAS PROSTATE CANCER

"Love never fails."

1 Cor. 13:8.

Looking back, that very first week after I was diagnosed is still vivid in my mind. It was the longest, hardest, and *loneliest* week I had to endure in my struggle with prostate cancer. Those were the seven days I withheld my terrible secret from everyone, including the person closest to me — my wife, Nancy.

Of course, Nancy could see something was wrong. I was withdrawn, morose, incommunicative — not at all my normal self, I assure you! Occasionally, concerns at work weigh on me, although rarely so visibly. However, because I prefer to solve work-related difficulties on my own, Nancy chose to wait and give me the opportunity to tell her what was bothering me on my own initiative.

With every passing day, I became more keenly aware of my need to tell Nancy about my diagnosis with prostate cancer. Intellectually, I realized that she had a right to know, for this problem would deeply affect her as well. But emotionally, I just wasn't ready.

When I could wait no longer, I revealed my secret. At first with apprehension and then with growing relief, I shared with Nancy what the doctor had found the week before. Just knowing she knew relieved some of the burden.

I was also pleased to see how well she took the news. She was clearly concerned, but expressed confidence that we would get through this calamity. At a time when I was suffering from many doubts and fears about my situation, this was a great encouragement.

My worst week was over, but for Nancy, the crisis was just beginning. Yet with the fallout of last week's news still clouding my mind, my own problems dominated my thoughts. After all, it occurred to me, she wasn't the one diagnosed with cancer ...

The Vicarious Victim

This observation reflects the common misconception that with cancer there is only one *real* casualty. Like most spouses, Nancy also assumed that because I was the one with cancer, I was the one in need of love and support. This same attitude is mirrored by health care providers, who tend to focus, sometimes exclusively, on the problems of the cancer patient. After all, the patient is the victim, right?

In the traditional view of the medical community and its support services, the nuclear family is seen primarily as a source of emotional support to those facing cancer. Certainly the afflicted individual is the only one that faces the bodily harm caused by cancer, and that ultimate of physical consequences, death. And certainly those closest to the patient can be of great value in providing comfort and support to the stricken individual.

But this should not lead us to diminish the cost to others. The devastation wrought by cancer does not stop with the cancer patient. It spreads to spouses, relatives, friends — in essence, everyone who knows and cares for the cancer sufferer. To a greater or lesser degree, they are all victims. Those closest to the cancer patient, physically and emotionally, suffer the greatest repercussions.

For a man with prostate cancer, there is usually one other principal victim of the disease: his wife. Prostate cancer can turn her life upside down much as his own. Children too — especially when young and still dependent on their parents — can be greatly victimized by their father's cancer. The emotional cost to them is often enormous. But parents are often able to act as a buffer between their children and the full impact of the disease. The man and his wife who find ways to bear the brunt of the burden can help to minimize the impact of the disease on their kids. In addition, because prostate cancer usually strikes men over the age of 60, in the majority of cases the children will be grown and out of the house. This doesn't mean they won't be affected. They will. But separate lives and separate addresses will shield them, and only the man with prostate cancer and his wife will remain to suffer the full impact of the disease.

For the wife, although there is no tumor within her body, her husband's prostate cancer does have a real and palpable presence in her life. Because of it, she too must face the gravest of questions: Will my husband die? Will my children lose their father? How will I live without him? How will I make ends meet? What can I do? And like her husband, she will at times undoubtedly wonder, "Why me?"

Her daily life will be irrevocably changed. Her accustomed duties and activities may be completely disrupted. She may find herself weighed down with new and unfamiliar responsibilities, as she faces the prospect of caring for and possibly supporting her husband during his treatment and possibly afterwards. With her husband, she must cope with the impact the disease may have on their marriage relationship — their sex life, their social life, and the way they interact together may all be dramatically altered. In so many ways, she is a partner to his pain.

Coping With The Pains Of Partnership

If your husband has prostate cancer, then you have firsthand experience with the pain of partnership. In chapter two of this book, *Fear and Trembling*, we talked about many of the emotional conflicts men face when confronted with prostate cancer, and ways to cope with these feelings. Your husband is experiencing many of these feelings now as he contends with the effects of his disease. Yet you too must endure the emotional turmoil that has come about as a consequence of your husband's prostate cancer. Although you may be experiencing many emotions similar to those of your husband, certain problems you must deal with are unique. How do you cope with your own feelings and emotions while providing support and encouragement to your husband?

This is the paradox you must resolve as the wife of the prostate cancer patient. Although you may suffer from the ravages of your husband's cancer as intensely as he does, you also find yourself thrust into the role of caretaker. In an effort to ease your husband's suffering, you may choose, as many wives do, to suffer in silence while making every effort to appear cheerful and optimistic. This approach may work occasionally, but often it will backfire. He may realize that you are not being open with him or treating him as an adult, adding to his feelings of isolation and helplessness. In addition, maintaining the facade will place additional strains on your marriage relationship, sometimes leading to increased conflict or breakdown. The well-being of your marriage is probably best served by finding a balance between your own emotional needs and the physical and emotional needs of your husband. Like all the troubles that couples face in life, the battle against prostate cancer is best undertaken as a partnership. Both you and your husband will be better off if you can work together as a team against the common enemy.

The following are some of the emotional problems that you may confront as a consequence of your husband's prostate cancer.

Fear

Cancer is always very frightening. Even the word is scary. Because you have almost as much to lose as your husband, it is to be expected that you will suffer a great deal of fear and anxiety. The idea of losing your loved one may be overwhelming. And your husband's fear may by sympathetic response intensify your own distress.

Sometimes the increased demands placed on you can be frightening, especially in the face of an uncertain future. You may feel inadequate to deal with all of your new responsibilities. Worry over your husband's condition may leave you troubled and distraught, anxious and uncertain about how to help him during this crisis. Confusion, moments of panic, and interrupted sleep patterns can all result from such chronic anxiety.

Fears are normal and unavoidable when cancer is involved. But if you find yourself struggling to keep your fears under control, there are things you can do to make your anxieties manageable:

• ***Realize that worrying won't make your husband any better.*** Excessive concern may cause you to become smothering and overprotective, or to "walk on pins and needles" to avoid doing anything to upset your husband. Although these behaviors are intended to relieve the strains your husband is going through, usually they will only add to them. On the other hand, indiscriminately pouring out all your anxieties on your husband is an unnecessary burden for him to bear. He has plenty of fears of his own. Try to treat him much as you normally would, but don't be afraid to gently express your concern for him. In this way, you can be a comfort to him, and hopefully he will respond in a way that will help to comfort your fears.

• ***Remember that prostate cancer is usually slow growing.*** Most men with prostate cancer do not die of the disease, and will usually live for years after diagnosis. You have time yet to be together. Making an effort to learn more about the disease may help to allay your fears.

• ***Share your fears with others.*** Merely talking to family members was a relief for Nancy. Simply knowing she didn't have to deal with her fears alone helped to alleviate them. Be cautious however with any family member you think may be unable to handle the news. Young children especially should not be overburdened with your fears since they are seldom equipped to deal with them.

• *Join a support group.* There are several support groups for those with cancer and their families. Man To Man and US TOO are both dedicated specifically to victims of prostate cancer (*see Appendix A: Where To Get Help*). Sympathetic strangers who understand what you are going through can be a great source of comfort — without the potential complications that can arise when family and friends are involved.

• *Keep yourself busy.* Do things that take your mind off your troubles. If you find yourself attending to your husband and his needs to the exclusion of all else, you should find some way to get away for a while. It will do both of you good.

• *Practice relaxation techniques.* Many individuals can help to reduce their tension level through the use of deep breathing exercises, progressive relaxation, and other relaxation techniques. In addition, a massage or warm bath can be very restful and soothing.

• *Pray.* Many people with spiritual convictions find solace through prayer and meditation. Nancy and I both found reliance on God a source of peace in times of trouble and uncertainty.

• *Take one day at a time.* Resist the urge to become fixated on what the unknowable future may hold. Take reasonable steps to prepare for any contingency, but keep your mind focused on the short-term. Similarly, keep your thoughts on those things over which you have some control, rather than things you cannot control, such as the results of your husband's diagnostic tests. In this way, you can maximize the help you can provide to your husband while minimizing the anxieties you must endure.

Anger

If you have experienced feelings of irrational anger directed at your husband since his diagnosis with prostate cancer, you are not the only one. Anger is an emotion many women have difficulty admitting to themselves, let alone to others. Our society deems anger an inappropriate emotion in women, so many women learn to repress feelings of hostility. The discomfort most women experience with anger may be particularly unsettling under circumstances such as these, when such feelings seem so inappropriate.

Do you find your temper flaring up unexpectedly, or feel a growing sense of resentment toward your husband? Perhaps it makes you feel guilty or ashamed to resent your husband in his hour of need. After all, you tell yourself, it isn't really his fault that he's sick.

But this resentment is a quite natural reaction to the additional frustrations of your situation. You may be longing for the way things were. But now, new duties, greater demands on your time, and yearnings that are frustrated have increased the stress of your daily life. He may not be doing what you think is necessary. Feelings of anger grow out of such conditions of increased tension.

Coping with anger is difficult, but it can be done. First of all, you need to admit to yourself that you really are angry. An inability to admit your inner anger can lead to far more destructive outlets for your anger. You may begin to feel more distant and indifferent toward your husband. You may turn on others besides your husband, or you may become deeply depressed and self-destructive. Far better than any of these is facing your anger and finding ways to overcome it.

To defuse your anger, recognize that its source is the increased stress of the situation, not your husband. If you have been experiencing more conflict with your husband, he too may be dealing with anger arising from frustration over his condition. Perhaps he is feeling uncustomarily helpless and dependent, and taking it out on you. Knowing this, direct your anger at the real source of frustration for both of you: the cancer itself. The best way to beat the enemy is to support your husband. Certainly he would gladly be rid of the cancer and release you from your additional duties if he could.

At the same time, find ways that you can release your tension and frustration. Do something that you enjoy. Go shopping, see a movie, visit a friend. Anything that reduces pent up energy will help you control feelings of anger. Crying is one common and effective way women sublimate feelings of anger they wish to avoid expressing in a more destructive way. Tears can be very therapeutic and stress-reducing. Incidentally, although a good cry may be a tremendous release for you, your husband might find it very upsetting. Try to find someplace away from him, so that you don't increase his stress while reducing your own.

You may feel that your anger is justified. Perhaps you feel you are bearing too much of the burden for your husband or others. If so, try to avoid venting your anger on your husband. Instead, talk with him calmly and gently (*see also Opening the Lines of Communication, on p. 194*). Remember what he is going through as well when you find yourself struggling to maintain your temper. You need support for yourself, too, so don't be ashamed to accept help from friends and family to relieve some of your burden.

Guilt

Feelings of guilt develop out of thoughts of failure and self-blame. Perhaps you feel you are not doing enough for your husband, or are failing to live up to your obligations. Do you feel a sudden aversion to your loved one, now that he has been diagnosed with cancer? Do you find yourself trying to avoid spending time with him? Resentment of your husband or the limitations his disease has imposed on your life may leave you feeling like a neglectful wife. Perhaps you feel ashamed at inappropriate thoughts that have come unexpectedly to your mind. You may even be blaming yourself for your husband's illness.

All of these things can lead to a sense of guilt. First, ask yourself what is at the root of your feelings of guilt. Have you done anything for which your conscience is bothering you? Are your guilty feelings exaggerated? You may have unrealistic expectations of yourself, in which case you need to come to an understanding of what you can and cannot do. One thing you cannot do is make your husband better, any more than you could have prevented his prostate cancer in the first place. Your love and support is important to your husband, but your constant attention is probably unwarranted. Indeed, he may be feeling guilty for the demands his condition is placing on you. For both your sakes, try to find a happy medium between caring for your husband and caring for your own well-being.

Many people experience aversion around sick individuals. If you do, remind yourself that although ill, your husband is the same man he always was. If his body has been affected by the disease, his spirit remains unchanged. Also keep in mind that his cancer is not contagious and cannot harm you in any way. Use your desire to be supportive as a weapon against these irrational feelings of aversion and the guilt they produce.

If you conclude that you have real reason to feel guilty, do something about it. Escape and avoidance are common but largely unproductive coping responses. If you respond to pressure by looking for an escape route, work on changing your response. Also seek ways to reduce the amount of pressure you feel. Even guilt can be used as an escape, so don't dwell on your guilt feelings. Instead, take positive actions to lessen the guilt you feel. When you feel like running away, try setting limited short-term goals that you feel confident you can accomplish. Don't get caught in an endless cycle of failure and self-condemnation.

Depression

Some degree of depression may be inescapable. That's okay. Along with your husband, you may experience many ups and downs during his treatment for prostate cancer. But when a period of discouragement slides into chronic depression, real problems can result. For this reason, it is important to overcome these natural periods of despondency should they show signs of persisting.

Depression can have wide-ranging effects. You may feel listless or exhausted, and unable to enjoy those things that normally bring you pleasure. Interacting with others may become a chore, and your daily tasks may suddenly seem too much to bear.

Perhaps the idea of your loved one's suffering and possible loss may be unutterably depressing to you. Changes in your life — difficult adjustments and altered plans — are also quite naturally a discouragement. And because prostate cancer can be a long-term problem, stretching into years, hopelessness may set in, threatening a deeper and more enduring state of despair.

Exerting the necessary effort to overcome your depression may seem depressing in and of itself! But it's worth it. First of all, examine yourself to see if any of the negative emotions described above are contributing to your depression. If so, take what steps you can to control and reduce those emotions.

Your depression may stem from an inability to express your true feelings. The drain of always trying to maintain a cheerful face for your husband's sake may be fueling your feelings of depression. Your attempts to steadfastly maintain a positive demeanor are not only unrealistic but may not be responsive to your husband's real needs. If he is sad and depressed, your apparent cheerfulness may leave him feeling isolated. He may even feel you don't really care about what is happening to him. But in reality grief is love experiencing loss. Thus, sharing your sorrow and grief together over your mutual losses can be an expression of love, and may provide a bridge out of despair for both of you.

Opening The Lines of Communication

Many patients learn the importance of open communication to establish a relationship of trust between patient and doctor. Similarly, honest and open expression between you and your husband is needed if the two of you are to successfully turn the resources of your marriage against the problems you confront. Sadly, much as a "conspiracy of silence" may mar the doctor-patient relationship, an atmosphere of secrecy may develop within a family or marriage when information is withheld from the patient "for his own good." In addition, the emotionally charged issues produced by prostate cancer can be extremely difficult to talk about. A married couple who have always maintained honest, intimate communication in their relationship may find that prostate cancer has created a wall of silence between them. Many marriages have never achieved the level of open communication that this situation demands of them. For these couples, the very idea of expressing the complex emotions they are experiencing may seem unimaginable.

Many times, each partner is afraid to say anything that might hurt the other. They try to protect each other by hiding the emotions they are feeling. It may seem easier and more comfortable that way. But at a time when they need each other most, a pattern of withholding leads both toward isolation. This can intensify their negative emotions and lead to exaggerated fears about what their partner is going through.

In such an atmosphere, both may come to feel as though they are living with a monster in their midst, yet are compelled to ignore its existence. The lack of communication between them undermines their ability to show love and support for each other. Only by bridging the widening gulf between them can their relationship become an instrument of healing and harmony.

Not every individual is able to express disturbing emotions, or talk about the frightening life-changes that emerge from a serious illness. No one should be compelled to talk against his or her will. In addition, there is no guarantee that every couple will successfully cope with all the new pressures on their relationship. The strain on some relationships can result in divisions in the marriage and professional counseling may be needed to save the relationship. But those couples that grow closer and stronger in such a crisis usually do so by striving to maintain honest and open communication.

When It's Time To Talk

The first steps toward openness are the most terrifying. No matter how well you know your husband, you are unlikely to know for sure how he will react. You may be afraid of losing control of your own emotions should you open up. Perhaps you simply don't know how to begin such a momentous conversation.

There is no easy set of rules to follow to develop good communication. People and their relationships differ. You will have to rely on a certain degree of intuition to know when is a good time for the two of you to talk.

Here are a few guidelines that may make it a little easier to open the lines of communication with your husband.

• *Give him time to adjust.* Everyone has his or her own emotional timetable for coming to terms with the impact of cancer. Like me, your husband may need a period of private introspection. Respect his privacy rather than trying to push him into a discussion of his illness before he is ready.

You too will probably need time to recover your emotional equilibrium. It's not uncommon for the spouse of a cancer sufferer to have a more difficult time coping with the disease than the patient. If you are having a hard time absorbing the shock of your partner's diagnosis, you may not feel ready to talk. You may be having trouble accepting the situation. If so, try not to shut him out or avoid him if he seeks to talk seriously with you. After all, it probably took considerable courage for him to risk initiating conversation about this sensitive issue. Express a willingness to talk with him, but request that he give you a little more time to digest the news. You may even suggest a day sometime in the near future when you will be ready to talk.

• *Prepare for sharing your concerns.* Try to put your feelings into words before talking with your husband. Do you identify with any of the emotional responses described in the previous section, *Coping With the Pains of Partnership?* What are your concerns regarding prostate cancer and its treatment? What questions do you have about what your husband is feeling or what you can do for him?

It may help you to clarify your concerns by writing down those things you would like to talk about with your partner. Talking through your feelings with another first may also help. This individual could be a friend, family member, or professional counselor. Or you might want to talk to someone who can better identify with your situation. There are several support groups and cancer hotlines that will allow you to speak directly to others who have experienced cancer firsthand (*see Appendix A: Where To Get Help*).

* *Let him choose the time to talk.* Your husband is the one most intimately affected by the cancer. For this reason, allow him to choose the moment to initiate discussion about his condition. The first words may be halting and brief — he may not say much at all — but that's all right. After all, you don't need to say everything immediately. Some things you may never need to say. What's important is that the door will have been opened.

In the meantime, you don't have to wait idly for your husband to break the silence. There are ways you can encourage openness. Indicate a readiness to listen, and show your support for him through your presence and continued attention to his needs. A touch, a hug, a loving gesture will let him know you are there for him. That way, when he is ready to talk, he will know you have a willing and sympathetic ear waiting for him.

• ***Look for cues.*** Just like you, your husband may not know how to begin. Watch for signs that he wants to talk, but is struggling to find the words. If you are usually the verbal initiator in your marriage relationship, he may be waiting for you to start. Awkwardness or nervousness in your presence, or talking around the subject, are usually good indications that he wants to talk openly. Even signs of irritation or open frustration may signal his desire to talk. He may use eye contact or a touch to reach out to you. Rely on your familiarity with your husband to sense when he is ready to talk, but waiting for you to make the first move.

• ***Continue to share.*** Initial conversations may reveal unexpected emotions in your partner. He may even direct his anger and frustration toward you. Don't let that keep you from sharing your concerns with him in the future. It may be unpleasant at times, but it is necessary. Remember that his negative feelings are really caused by the cancer, not by you.

Through the ups and downs of therapy, open communication may lapse. Disappointment or resentment may be hindering openness. This can happen in any marriage, regardless of the circumstances. However, this is not a good time to stop talking with each other. Communication won't bring an easy resolution to the problems you and your husband face, but it will allow you to face those problems together.

The Home Front

In the war on prostate cancer, the weapons are wielded by physicians. The scalpel, the linear accelerator, the radioisotope, the pill, the injection: these are the weapons of destruction in this war. When the cancer is killed, the war is won.

But the fact that you're not on the front lines of the battle shouldn't minimize your role in winning this war. You represent the home front. You work to keep morale high.

Just as women in wartime may have felt helpless as they watched filmrolls of their men overseas, you may have feelings of helplessness. But your job is a vital one, and there are many things you can do to help your husband win this war. Here are some of the things you can do to make a difference.

Create a Comforting Environment

For most men, home is their refuge from troubles. But cancer brings trouble to his home. Changed roles and family upheaval may turn his household into a stressful environment.

Make every effort to open up communication so that a conspiratorial atmosphere does not develop. When necessary, work with your husband to reorganize family responsibilities so as to make the transition as smooth as possible. Your spouse may feel despondent if he has been suddenly thrust into a state of dependence. While remaining sensitive to his feelings, focus on immediate problems in a pragmatic way. Let him know these changes are just temporary and for the sake of expedience.

Keep everyday life on an even keel. Try to maintain your family's regular routine. A sense of the familiar at home will help compensate for the chaos that has entered your husband's life.

Learn With Him

Show interest in your husband and his problem by joining him in learning about prostate cancer, its implications and treatment. What you learn will help you understand better what your husband is up against. At the same time, you can encourage your husband to become better informed.

After I told Nancy about my prostate cancer, she took me by the hand and we headed over to the local bookstore. This started me on the way toward taking charge of what was happening to me. Education is a great antidote for the sense of helplessness cancer can create, in both you and your husband. And as it did for me, it may reveal a solution to your husband's problem he did not know existed.

Support His Treatment Decisions

Along with learning more about prostate cancer at home, you can accompany your husband when he has an appointment see his physician. Don't insist if he does not want you to come. However, in most cases, he will be glad for the additional support.

Although you may feel pushy, be sure to ask questions about anything of concern to you. The physician may not know what is important to you, or may feel uncomfortable revealing certain information until asked. And because physicians are busy people, they may not even realize that they have left out certain details. Questions about treatments and their side-effects, medications, nutrition, physical and emotional problems: all are appropriate. Writing questions down before seeing the doctor is a good idea. Be sensitive to your husband's feelings if he is present during your questioning. You may want to talk to the doctor separately about certain issues. If you do, avoid hiding information from your husband that he has a right to know.

Feel free to talk with your partner about various treatments and their possible complications. Let him know your concerns. However, when it comes time to choose a medical treatment, you may have to leave the final decision to him. It is his body, and ultimately his life.

This may be very difficult at times. Nancy felt strongly that the radical prostatectomy was the best way to go. She was concerned about the relatively new nature of the treatment I chose. Although she found this frustrating, she ultimately supported my decision.

If you feel very strongly that your spouse is making a poor decision, and constructive discussion has not changed his mind, further dispute is unlikely to do any good. If you believe it might sway his decision, you could ask him to talk with a professional, a physician or counselor who could advise him. If this should fail, let him know that even though you disagree with his choice, you respect his right to choose. Then stand by him.

Keep Him Involved

He is almost certain to experience some degree of isolation. The impact of cancer on your partner's life may cause him to withdraw. He may not be physically able to do some of the things he did before. His work or usual activities may no longer be available outlets for him. And because so many people find it uncomfortable to be around someone with cancer, he may sense the outside world withdrawing from him.

Because you are closest to him, make an effort to act as a connection between him and the outside world. At times you may be so busy that you find yourself leading a separate life from him. If so, try to arrange your schedule in order to spend time together and involve him in your life. Keep in contact with friends and relatives, and urge them to call or visit. Encourage your husband to remain as active as he can, without pushing him to doing anything he truly doesn't feel up to doing. He may need some responsible pursuits to keep life purposeful. And without fun and recreation, life becomes dreary.

Pain, fatigue and depression may be interfering with your husband's ability to remain active. See what you can do to mitigate these debilitating influences. Join him in finding creative alternatives to the things that are now missing from his life. With a little effort, you can find positive ways for your partner to stay involved.

Help Him to Help Himself

Chapter 9, *Fitness, Diet, and Nutrition,* discusses some of the ways that a man with prostate cancer can take action to improve his condition. You can be a vital aid in any self-help program he chooses to undertake. Design a menu that provides good nutrition and takes advantage of our current knowledge about the health-promoting powers of certain foods. Naturally, you shouldn't deny him the occasional indulgence in foods he enjoys, or force him to eat what he doesn't like. Even smoking shouldn't be denied him if he wants to continue. If he does not want to quit, encourage him to cut back. Remember that these changes in his lifestyle are made because they have been statistically shown to provide an advantage in cancer prevention and treatment. Even so, they alone cannot determine whether he will recover from prostate cancer or not. In fact, robbing him of his pleasures may only serve to lower his spirits, which might counteract any good that would otherwise result from healthy lifestyle changes.

Your loving support can also help your husband fight off the emotional effects of prostate cancer. This doesn't mean you always have to be up and energetic around him. Sometimes, commiserating with him over your struggles together will let him know someone shares in his suffering. Talk with him often so you can better understand how he is feeling, and how you can help. Rather than giving him false hope, try to find ways to inspire real hopefulness in him. Your hopeful attitude can work to revitalize his own sense of optimism.

Reassure Him of His Manhood

Many of the consequences of prostate cancer and its treatments can undermine your husband's feelings of masculinity. He may also no longer be able to assume the traditional male role in the family. Loss of energy and changes in physical appearance can make him seem less robust. Certain drugs used to treat prostate cancer may also make him appear less manly, particularly to himself. The most profound change of all may be his loss of sexual desire or ability, a relatively common complication of therapy for prostate cancer.

As a result, your husband's sense of manhood may be at an all-time low. Like many wives, you may be most concerned about the physical welfare of your husband. Consequently, you may not fully appreciate the terrible pain this attack on his virility is causing your mate.

There are several things you can do to help avert the catastrophic loss of self-esteem that may result. Let him know that your love for him is not a consequence of his physical characteristics but of his personal qualities, which remain unchanged. And though his body image might have suffered, even little things like getting his help opening a jar or bringing in the groceries may bolster his sense of masculinity. Most of all, physical contact will indicate your continued affection for him. Try to tell your partner through touch or word that physical closeness with him remains important to you. Hugging, cuddling and caressing will reassure your husband that you find him desirable, and will be a comfort to you as well.

Showing affection for your husband may sound simple, but sometimes nothing could be harder, especially if you are feeling less desirable because he is no longer approaching you. But physical withdrawal from each other will only make it more difficult to restore closeness later on. Finding a support group with others that share these problems may be a great help to both of you.

If the prostate cancer has impacted your sexual relationship with your husband, explore ways in which you and your partner can change your expression of sexual interest in each other (*see Overcoming The Threat To Intimacy,* on p. 171).

Give Him Your Love

Love is the greatest gift you can give to your husband. There is a reason we always hear about the magical quality that love possesses: because it is true. I know from my own experience that the power of love to heal and restore is immeasurable.

Love is also the fundamental reason for your desire to help your husband. While you are busy doing those things mentioned above, take the time to remind him why. Reminders of your love can ease his burdens, and make life worth living. In this way, you can do for him what no one else can. Of all the things you do on his behalf, put loving him at the top of your list.

Where To Get Help

A trusted physician who is familiar with the particular details of your case should be your first and foremost source of information and advice. Nonetheless, for those who desire additional information, there are a number of organizations dedicated to helping patients and their families cope with prostate cancer. These agencies not only provide information and counseling, but in some cases may provide financial aid and transportation to a medical facility for treatment.

The following is a list of national organizations that provide information and services for prostate cancer patients. Each entry gives the current address and phone number, programs sponsored by the organization, and a brief description.

For information on local support groups, contact the social service office of a local hospital, or write or call one of the national cancer information services that follow.

American Cancer Society (ACS)

1599 Clifton Road, N.E.
Atlanta, GA 30329
(800) ACS-2345

CanSurmount
I Can Cope
Man To Man Prostate Cancer Support Groups

The American Cancer Society is involved in education and research, and offers counseling and other patient services. The Society consists of 3000 local chapters across the United States, and has recently adopted the Man to Man prostate cancer support group program on a national basis.

American Foundation of Urologic Disease

300 West Pratt Street,
Suite 401
Baltimore, MD 21201-2463
(800) 242-2383

US TOO Support Groups
Prostate Health Council

A nonprofit organization that provides education to the public, patients, and health care professionals about urologic diseases, with an emphasis on prostate cancer.

Cancer Information Service (CIS)

National Cancer Institute (NCI)
Building 31, Room 10A24
9000 Rockville Pike
Bethesda, MD 20892
(800) 4-CANCER

A governmental service that provides information over the telephone to cancer patients, the public, and health care professionals. Trained staff members can provide information on current treatments, cancer prevention, and the nearest Comprehensive Cancer Center. The National Cancer Institute also supplies a wide variety of written materials to answer questions about cancer. The PDQ, or Physician Data Query, is a computer information system that provides doctors and patients with the latest information on clinical trials and their results. The Cancer Information Service will provide a copy of the PDQ to anyone who requests it.

Corporate Angel Network (CAN)

Westchester County Airport Building 1
White Plains, NY 10604
(914) 328-1313

A service that provides volunteer corporate aircraft for those in need of transportation between home and a cancer treatment center.

Help for Incontinent People

P.O. Box 8306
Spartanburg, SC 29305
(800) BLADDER

A nonprofit organization that provides information and other services to those suffering from incontinence problems. Help for Incontinent People produces the *HIP Report,* a quarterly newsletter that gives written responses to questions about incontinence.

Impotence Institute of America

2020 Pennsylvania Ave. NW, Suite 292
Washingtion DC 20006
(800) 669-1603

Impotence Anonymous

A nonprofit organization dedicated to helping men with impotence problems and their partners. The Institute provides information and physician referrals, and is sponsor of Impotence Anonymous, a support group with chapters in most major metropolitan centers.

Make Today Count

c/o Connie Zimmerman
Mid-America Cancer Center
1235 E. Cherokee
Springfield, MO 65804-2263
(800) 432-2273

Provides counseling and emotional support to those with advanced cancer and their families. There are several hundred local chapters in the United States.

Man To Man

c/o American Cancer Society
1599 Clifton Road, N.E.
Atlanta, GA 30329
(800) ACS-2345

Man To Man is a national support group officially sponsored by the American Cancer Society to provide information and support to men with prostate cancer and their families. To find out more about Man To Man, contact the American Cancer Society at the address and phone number listed above.

The Mathews Foundation For Prostate Cancer Research

1010 Hurley Way, Suite 195
Sacramento, CA 95825
(800) 234-6284

The Mathews Foundation is committed to expanding public awareness of prostate cancer, funding research into the genetic causes of prostate cancer, and providing information and one-on-one counseling to prostate cancer patients and their families through their national toll-free hotline.

Patient Advocates for Advanced Cancer Treatments (PAACT)

1143 Parmelee NW
Grand Rapids, MI 49504
(616) 453-1477

A nonprofit organization for both patients and physicians that promotes an understanding of prostate cancer, its diagnosis and therapeutic treatment. PAACT has a database on over 14,500 men with prostate cancer, and readily provides information concerning alternative treatments by telephone to those diagnosed with prostate cancer.

Theragenics Corporation

5325 Oak Brook Parkway
Norcross, GA 30093
(800) 458-4372

Theragenics is the manufacturer of the radio-active palladium seeds used in brachytherapy for the treatment of prostate cancer. The company readily supplies information to those interested in knowing more about the seed implantation procedure and Theragenics' products.

US TOO Support Groups

US TOO, Inc.
P.O. Box 7173
Oak Brook Terrace, IL 60181
(800) 82-US-TOO

The mission of US TOO, a support group sponsored by the American Foundation for Urologic Disease, is to provide counseling, fellowship, and support to cancer patients and their families. Contact the national headquarters of US TOO at the address and number above to find out where the nearest US TOO chapter is located.

GLOSSARY OF MEDICAL TERMS

Adenocarcinoma. A cancer originating in glandular tissue. Prostate cancer is classified as adenocarcinoma of the prostate.

Adjuvant. An additional treatment used to increase the effectiveness of the primary therapy. Radiation therapy and hormonal therapy are often used as adjuvant treatments following a radical prostatectomy.

Analog. A man-made chemical compound that is structurally similar to one produced naturally by the body. *See LHRH analogs.*

Androgen. A hormone that produces male characteristics. *See testosterone.*

Anesthetic. A drug that produces general or local loss of physical sensations, particularly pain.

A "spinal" is the injection of a local anesthetic into the area surrounding the spinal cord.

Antiandrogen. A drug that blocks the activity of androgens produced by the adrenal glands at the cellular receptor sites.

Antibody. A protein produced by the body that counteracts the toxic effects of a foreign substance, organism, or disease within the body.

Benign. A non-cancerous condition. *See Benign Prostatic Hypertrophy.*

Benign Prostatic Hypertrophy. Also Benign Prostatic Hyperplasia, or BPH. A non-cancerous condition of the prostate that results in a growth of tumorous tissue and increase in the size of the prostate.

Biopsy. A procedure involving the removal of tissue from the body of the patient. Removed tissue is typically examined microscopically by a pathologist in order to make a precise diagnosis of the patient's condition.

BPH. See Benign Prostatic Hypertrophy.

Brachytherapy. A form of radiation therapy in which radioactive seeds are implanted into the prostate to deliver radiation directly to the tumor.

Cancer. A cellular malignancy typically forming tumors. Unlike benign tumors, these tend to invade surrounding tissues and spread to distant sites of the body.

Carcinoma. A malignant tumor made up chiefly of epithelial cells, or those cells that form the lining of an organ or cavity. *See Adenocarcinoma.*

Chemotherapy. The treatment of cancer using chemicals that deter the growth of cancer cells.

Combination Therapy. A form of hormonal therapy that surgically or chemically blocks the production of testosterone by the testes, and involves the additional use of an antiandrogen to block the receptor sites from utilizing testosterone produced by the adrenal glands.

Conformal. A treatment conforming precisely to the size and shape of the prostate, with the use of computerized planning and state-of-the-art imaging techniques.

Cryosurgery. The freezing of tissue with the use of liquid nitrogen probes. When used to treat prostate cancer, the cryoprobes are guided by transrectal ultrasound.

Diagnosis. Evaluation of a patient's symptoms and/or test results, with the intent of identifying and verifying the existence of any underlying disease or abnormal condition.

Digital Rectal Examination (DRE). A procedure in which the physician inserts a gloved, lubricated finger into the rectum to examine the prostate gland for signs of cancer.

Ejaculatory Ducts. The tubular passages through which semen reaches the prostatic urethra during orgasm.

Erectile Dysfunction. *See impotence.*

Estrogen. A female sex hormone, used as a form of therapy to inhibit the production of testosterone in patients diagnosed with prostate cancer.

False Negative. An erroneous negative test result. For example, an imaging test that fails to show the presence of a cancer tumor later found by biopsy to be present in the patient is said to have returned a false negative result.

False Positive. A positive test result mistakenly identifying a state or condition that does not in fact exist.

Frozen Section. A technique in which removed tissue is frozen, cut into thin slices, and stained for microscopic examination. A pathologist can rapidly complete a frozen section analysis, and for this reason, it is commonly used during surgery to quickly provide the surgeon with vital information.

Gland. An aggregation of cells that secretes a substance for use or discharge from the body.

Gleason Score. A widely used method for classifying the cellular differentiation of cancerous tissue. The less the cancerous cells appear like normal cells, the more malignant the cancer. Two grades of 1-5, identifying the two most common degrees of differentiation present in the examined tissue sample, are added together to produce the Gleason score.

Gynecomastia. A side effect of some forms of hormonal therapy, involving breast growth and tenderness.

Hormonal therapy. Cancer treatment involving the blockage of hormone production by surgical or chemical means. Because prostate cancer is usually dependent on male hormones to grow, hormonal therapy can be an effective means of alleviating symptoms and retarding the development of the disease.

Impotence. The loss of ability to produce and/or sustain an erection.

Incontinence. A loss of urinary control. There are various kinds and degrees of incontinence. *Overflow incontinence* is a condition in which the bladder retains urine after voiding. As a consequence, the bladder remains full most of the time, resulting in involuntary seepage of urine from the bladder. *Stress incontinence* is the involuntary discharge of urine when there is increased pressure upon the bladder, as in coughing or straining to lift heavy objects. *Total incontinence* is the failure of ability to voluntarily exercise control over the sphincters of the bladder neck and urethra, resulting in total loss of retentive ability.

Inflammation. Redness or swelling caused by injury or infection.

Informed Consent. Permission to proceed given by a patient after being fully informed of the purposes and potential consequences of a medical procedure.

Investigational. A drug or procedure allowed by the FDA for use in clinical trials.

Laparoscopic Lymphadenectomy. The removal of pelvic lymph nodes with a laparoscope via four small incisions in the lower abdomen.

LHRH Analogs. Synthetic compounds that are chemically similar to Luteinizing Hormone

Releasing Hormone (LHRH), used to suppress tes-ticular production of testosterone.

Luteinizing Hormone Releasing Hormone (LHRH). A hormone that regulates the production of sex hormones in men and women.

Lymphadenectomy. The removal and examination of lymph nodes to precisely diagnose and stage cancer.

Lymph Node. A small bean-shaped mass of tissue along the vessels of the lymphatic system. The lymph nodes filter out bacteria and other toxins, as well as cancer cells.

Malignant. Tending to become progresssively worse and to result in death. Having the invasive and metastatic properties of cancer.

Metastasis. The spread of cancer, by way of the blood stream or lymphatic system, beyond the boundaries of the organ or structure where the cancer originated. *Metastases* is the plural.

Metastatic Work Up. A group of tests, including bone scans, x-rays, and blood tests, to ascertain whether cancer has metastasized.

Morbidity. Unhealthy consequences and complications resulting from treatment.

Oncology. The branch of medical science dealing with tumors. An oncologist is a specialist in the study of cancerous tumors.

Orchiectomy. A simple operation that involves surgical removal of the testicles, which produce most of the body's testosterone.

PAP. *See Prostatic Acid Phosphatase.*

Pathologist. A doctor who specializes in the examination of cells and tissues removed from the body.

Perineum. The area of the body between the anus and scrotum. A perineal procedure uses this area as the point of entry into the body.

Prognosis. A forecast of the course of a disease, and future prospects of the patient.

Progression. A change in the status of the cancer indicating the condition has progressed and worsened.

Prostate Specific Antigen (PSA). A blood test that measures a substance manufactured solely by prostate gland cells. An elevated reading indicates an abnormal condition of the prostate gland, either benign or malignant. It is presently the most sensitive tumor marker for the identification and monitoring of prostate cancer.

Prostatic Acid Phosphatase (PAP). An enzyme produced by the prostate that is elevated in many patients when prostate cancer has spread beyond the prostate.

PSA. *See Prostate Specific Antigen.*

Radiation Therapy. Use of high energy rays to kill cancer cells.

Radical Prostatectomy. An operation to remove the entire prostate gland and seminal vesicles.

Radio sensitivity. The degree to which a type of cancer responds to radiation therapy.

Recurrence. Return of the cancer following remission or treatment intended as curative. Local recurrence indicates a return of the cancer at the site of origin. Distant recurrence indicates the appearance of one or more metastases of the disease.

Refractory. A term indicating that the cancer no longer responds to the current therapy. *See progression.*

Remission. Complete or partial disappearance of the signs and symptoms of the disease. The period during which a disease remains under control, without progressing. Even complete remission does not necessarily indicate cure.

Stage. A term used to describe the extent of the disease. *See Staging, Whitmore-Jewett Staging.*

Staging. The testing process by which the extent and severity of a known cancer is evaluated according to an established system of classification. It is used to help determine appropriate therapy. *See Whitmore-Jewett Staging.*

Testosterone. A male sex hormone chiefly produced by the testicles.

Transurethral Resection of the Prostate (TURP). A surgical procedure to remove tissue obstructing the urethra. The technique involves the insertion of an instrument called a resectoscope into the penile urethra, and is intended to relieve obstruction of urine flow due to enlargement of the prostate.

Tumor. An excessive growth of cells caused by uncontrolled and disorderly cell replacement. *See Benign, Malignant.*

TURP. *See Transurethral Resection of the Prostate.*

Urethra. The tube that carries urine from the bladder and semen from the prostate out of the body through the penis.

Whitmore-Jewett Staging. A classification system for evaluating the extent of prostate cancer. Stages A-D are followed by numerical prefixes 1-3, indicating substages. This system is widely used for the designation of stage.

QUESTIONS TO ASK YOUR DOCTOR

Any man who has been told he has prostate cancer knows the feeling of shock that this diagnosis engenders. At first, this news will be all the patient can handle. But on a later visit, it is important to get further information from the diagnosing physician. The questions listed below will help the patient get a better understanding of his condition, and give him a foundation for preparing to deal with his prostate cancer.

- How do you know I have prostate cancer?

- Are there further tests I should have to determine the stage and nature of the cancer before I decide on a course of treatment? What will these tests tell us?

- What stage of prostate cancer do I have? How certain are you that my cancer is this stage?

- What are the alternative treatments for my stage of prostate cancer?

- Are there any treatment alternatives other than those you have mentioned?

- What are the risks involved in each of the various treatments?

- What would be the likely consequence of receiving no treatment?

- Will these treatments require hospitalization, or can they be performed on an outpatient basis?

- What do the different tests and treatments cost?

- What treatment do you recommend for me, and why?

- How many times have you performed this treatment in the last year?

- With the treatment you recommend, what is the *rate and degree* of impotence and incontinence among your patients?

- Does the site of the tumor in my prostate increase the risk of impotence or incontinence from the treatment you recommend?

- Is computerized planning sometimes involved in this treatment? Do you use such planning techniques? If not, why not?

- How will I feel during and after treatment?

- When will I be able to return to normal, everyday activities?

- When will I be able to resume sexual relations?

- What should I do if I experience impotence problems after treatment? Can you advise me or send me to someone who is an expert in the field?

- What should I do if I experience problems with incontinence after treatment? What can be done to treat incontinence? Is there an expert in the field you can refer me to in such an event?

- Will I need regular checkups to monitor the cancer and my response to treatment?

- What tests will be required for these checkups, and what will they tell us?

- Are there particular warning signs for problems I should be aware of relating to a worsening of my condition or that might result from treatment?

- Where should I go to get a second opinion?

DIAGNOSTIC AND STAGING TESTS

BIOPSY OF THE PROSTATE. The removal of a tissue sample from the prostate for microscopic examination. The biopsy is necessary to positively identify the presence of prostate cancer.

BONE SCAN. An imaging technique used to detect bone metastates, which appear as "hot spots" on the film. It is far more sensitive than the conventional x-ray.

COMPUTED TOMOGRAPHY (CT) SCAN. This sophisticated technique produces a 3-D x-ray image of the prostate gland and surrounding tissues. The CT scan can identify prostate enlargement, but is not always effective for assessing the stage of prostate cancer. For evaluating metastases of the lymph nodes or more distant soft tissue sites, the CT scan is significantly more accurate.

INTRAVENOUS PYELOGRAM (IVP). An x-ray which involves the injection of a special dye to check for the spread of cancer to the kidneys and bladder.

LYMPHADENECTOMY. Also known as a pelvic lymph node dissection, this procedure involves the removal and microscopic examination of selected lymph nodes, a common site of metastatic disease with prostate cancer. This procedure can be performed during surgery prior to the removal of the prostate gland, or a laparoscopic lymphadenectomy may by performed, a simple operation requiring only an overnight stay in the hospital.

MAGNETIC RESONANCE IMAGING (MRI). A state-of-the-art technique that generates a magnetic field, which harmlessly reacts with the tissues of the body to produce a distinct and complex image of internal organs. The MRI is primarily of use in staging biopsy-proven prostate cancer.

PROSTATE SPECIFIC ANTIGEN (PSA) TEST. An inexpensive blood test that measures the level of a protein typically found only in the prostate. The test can be used for the early detection of prostate cancer, as well as a means for estimating the extent of the disease. The PSA test is also a valuable tool for monitoring a patient's progress following treatment.

PROSTATIC ACID PHOSPHATASE (PAP) TEST. A blood test primarily used to check for the spread of prostate cancer to distant sites of the body. Its use has declined following the development of the more sensitive PSA test.

ULTRASOUND. Technically referred to as Transrectal Ultrasonography, this imaging technique projects sound waves off the prostate and surrounding organs to create an image. Ultrasound can in most cases accurately identify the local spread of prostate cancer, and is often used to guide biopsy of suspicious sites in the prostate.

INDEX

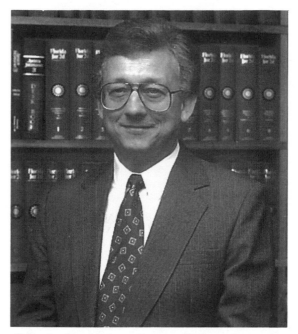

Don Kaltenbach at his law offices in New Port Richey, Florida.

About the Authors

Don Kaltenbach lives in New Port Richey with his wife, Nancy, and their three children, David, Graham, and Whitney, where he has practiced law for over twenty years. A prostate cancer survivor, Don often speaks to groups about his experience with prostate cancer, and counsels men who have been diagnosed with the disease.

Tim Richards is a freelance writer and editor who resides in Port Richey, Florida. He is co-author of the *Revell Bible Dictionary* and *It Couldn't Just Happen.*

To order more copies of *Prostate Cancer: A Survivor's Guide,* write or call:

Seneca House Press
Prostate Cancer Guide
P.O. Box 966
New Port Richey, FL 34656

(800) 915-1001